TODAY'S TREATMENT: 4

TODAY'S TREATMENT: 4

Articles published in
the *British Medical Journal*

Published by the British Medical Association
Tavistock Square, London WC1H 9JR

ISBN 0 7279 0076 5

Made and printed in England by
The Devonshire Press
Barton Road, Torquay

Preface

by the Editor

British Medical Journal

Britain spent more than one billion pounds on drugs in 1980, and more than three-quarters of the drugs were prescribed in general practice. Modern drugs are potent, dangerous, and expensive, and every doctor should have some knowledge of clinical pharmacology—a subject that has been badly taught in many medical schools. This fourth book in the series *Today's Treatment* contains a series of straightforward articles that serve as an invaluable introduction to this fast-changing discipline. Further articles discuss the increasingly important subject of drug-induced disease and others cover all the important topics in a discipline that depends heavily on drugs—anaesthetics. All the articles have been taken from the *BMJ* and have incorporated suggestions and criticisms made in the correspondence columns; they are thus both accurate and clear.

STEPHEN LOCK

March, 1981

Contents

Drug-induced diseases

Contents

Contents

Clinical Pharmacology

Contents

Drug-induced cardiovascular disease

ALASDAIR M BRECKENRIDGE

Adverse reactions to any group of drugs can be divided into those that occur as an exaggerated but otherwise normal response to the drug and those that represent aberrant effects unrelated to its therapeutic action. This review of drug-induced cardiovascular disease will deal principally with the second type of adverse reaction and will not discuss, in any depth, problems such as postural hypotension caused by antihypertensive agents, clinically important as they may be. In any survey of drug-induced disease cardiovascular drugs are among the commonest agents incriminated. The most frequent drug-induced cardiovascular disorders are probably cardiac arrhythmias, heart failure, changes in blood pressure, and vascular spasm.

DRUG-INDUCED ARRHYTHMIAS

Paradoxically, the commonest drugs to cause cardiac arrhythmias are those that are themselves used to treat rhythm disturbances. Although the incidence of digitalis-induced arrhythmias has decreased because of the wider use of potent diuretics in treating heart failure, these are still a source of concern, especially in elderly patients and those with compromised renal function. Virtually every type of arrhythmia, both ventricular and supraventricular, has been described with digitalis. The most worrying are ventricular ectopics occurring in runs, which may merge into short bursts of ventricular tachycardia or fibrillation. Even atrial fibrillation, itself an indication for digitalis treatment, may be a sign of overdosage. As with any other suspected digitalis-induced arrhythmias, drug withdrawal is advisable, and potassium should be replaced when necessary. If life threatening the arrhythmia should be treated with the appropriate agent, such as a beta-adrenoceptor blocking agent, disopyramide or phenytoin for tachycardia, and atropine for bradycardia.

Quinidine, phenytoin, procainamide, and, less often, lignocaine may also induce disorders of cardiac rhythm, as may sympathomimetic agents such as adrenaline, noradrenaline, and isoprenaline. The latter are often used for their chronotropic or inotropic action on the heart, but arrhythmias may occur when they are being used for a non-cardiac indication. Adrenaline, given as a vasoconstrictor with local anaesthetics, may be absorbed in sufficient quantities from vascular tissues to cause ectopic beats. The excessive death rate in young asthmatic patients recorded in the late 1960s has been attributed to the overuse of inhalers containing isoprenaline. Death was often sudden and unexpected, supporting the theory that an arrythmia due to the sympathomimetic agent may have been the precipitating event in an already hypoxaemic patient. Fluoroalkane gases in the propellant of the inhaler that sensitise the myocardium to the action of the sympathomimetic agent may also have played a part. Halothane may lead to ventricular arrhythmias due to its ability to sensitise the myocardium to catecholamines, either endogenously produced or exogenously administered. Halothane has, in addition, a direct vagal effect, which results in cardiac slowing, and this may be seen during induction of anaesthesia.

Centrally acting drugs with pronounced cardiovascular effects include tricyclic antidepressants, which by virtue of their anticholinergic effect pose problems of cardiac rhythm when taken in overdosage. Arrhythmias caused by phenothiazines, such as chlorpromazine, have a similar basis. The management of patients poisoned with overdoses of tricyclics or phenothiazines is difficult, and their prognosis often depends on the ability to prevent or control disorders of cardiac rhythm.

DEPRESSION OF CARDIAC FUNCTION

Heart failure resulting from administration of beta-adrenoceptor blocking drugs is an example of an exaggerated but otherwise normal drug response. In patients whose myocardial function is preserved only by virtue of a high level of adrenergic drive—that is, after cardiac surgery or in patients in incipient heart failure—administration of beta-blockers can precipitate frank decompensation, accompanied by bradycardia and hypotension. Intravenous administration of beta-blockers to treat a cardiac arrhythmia is not infrequently the precipitating cause. If beta-blockers must be given to patients with incipient failure by either oral or parenteral routes they should be administered very circumspectly and should be covered with digitalis. If heart failure is going to occur the first doses of beta-blockers will usually precipitate this, and thus it is always advisable to start with a low dose for one or two days before building up to an appropriate therapeutic regimen. The bradycardia produced by beta-blockers can be reversed initially by atropine given intravenously to oppose vagal effects. Isoprenaline will antagonise the adverse cardiac effects of beta-blockade on a competitive basis, but large doses may be needed.

Quinidine, procainamide, and lignocaine can all precipitate heart failure and hypotension by depressing myocardial excitability and prolonging the refractory period of cardiac muscle. These effects are dose dependent, and again are usually more evident with intravenously administered drugs, when a relatively larger proportion of the dose is distributed to the heart than when the drugs are given by mouth.

DRUG-INDUCED DISORDERS OF HEART MUSCLE

It is now well established that alcohol may exert a direct toxic effect on heart muscle, independent of the nutritional type of cardiomyopathy (akin to beri-beri) that alcoholics can suffer because of their poor diet. In this "direct" type of alcoholic cardiomyopathy the previous diet may have been quite adequate and replacement of thiamine is without effect. These patients present in heart failure with or without cardiac arrhythmias, and although conventional measures of treating failure at first meet with some success, the overall course is often progressive and downhill. Withdrawal of alcohol (even when possible) is no guarantee of a good outcome. Apparent "epidemics" of heart failure in beer drinkers in the United States were traced to the addition of cobalt to beer to produce a better "head." The death rate from heart failure in these outbreaks was high, but on withdrawal of the cobalt from beer no new cases were seen.

Cardiomyopathy is a well-recorded toxic sign of the antineoplastic agents, daunorubicin and its structural analogue, doxorubicin (Adriamycin). These effects are cumulative dose dependent; the drugs are taken up by the myocardial cells, and at necropsy a striking decrease in the number of cardiac cells can be seen together with degeneration of those remaining. Monitoring of the electrocardiogram and systolic time interval are probably the earliest predictors of toxicity, although awareness by the doctor that these drugs can cause heart failure is the best safeguard.

Experimental animal studies have shown that infusion of catecholamines at high doses can induce areas of myocardial necrosis and focal degeneration—a similar picture is occasionally seen in patients with phaeochromocytoma. These changes appear unlikely to occur with therapeutic doses of sympathomimetic agents, but they can be important in overdosage. Post-mortem changes of myofibrillary degeneration have been seen in patients given long-term high-dose phenothiazine treatment. The basis of this is uncertain, but it has been speculatively associated with the ability of phenothiazines to block catecholamine tissue uptake thus leading to high circulatory catecholamine concentrations.

Cardiomyopathy has also been occasionally found after lithium treatment, and this may become more of a problem as its use increases. More frequent are the abnormalities of cardiac function caused by emetine, used to treat amoebiasis. ECG changes such as T-wave inversion are extremely common, and it is now recommended that everyone given emetine is kept in bed during treatment, and for a few days after. Experimental animal work suggests that these cardiac effects of emetine are caused by its ability to inhibit cardiac protein biosynthesis.

Drug-induced cardiovascular disease

DRUGS CAUSING MYOCARDIAL ISCHAEMIA

Coronary artery disease is relatively infrequent in young women, and is at least six times more common in men between 30 and 54 than in women of the same age. Studies such as those carried out by the Royal College of General Practitioners have clearly indicated contraceptive steroids as a precipitating factor in myocardial ischaemia. The incidence of coronary artery and cerebrovascular disease is higher in pill users than those using other methods of contraception, and this is compounded by other factors, such as increasing age, smoking, obesity, and hypertension. The importance of increases in clotting factor concentrations induced by contraceptive steroids as a cause of vascular disease is uncertain, and other changes such as those in blood pressure and plasma lipids must also contribute.

Much effort has gone into examining the association between excessive coffee drinking and myocardial ischaemia; but on current available evidence a causal relation is hard to sustain.

DRUG-INDUCED HYPERTENSION

Most drugs that cause a chronic rise in blood pressure do so by causing retention of salt and water. Commonest examples are corticosteroids, contraceptive steroids, carbenoxolone, and phenylbutazone. Corticosteroids such as prednisone vary in their sodium retaining ability in patients, and this is paralleled by the variability in the levels of blood pressure in patients with Cushing's syndrome, but death from malignant hypertension has resulted from prolonged corticosteroid treatment. The precise pharmacological basis of contraceptive steroid-induced hypertension is uncertain, but it is now accepted that they cause an average increase of some 4 mm Hg systolic and 2 mm Hg diastolic blood pressure a year. Obviously in some patients the increase is greater, and again, cases of contraceptive-induced malignant hypertension have been reported. Withdrawal of contraceptive steroids does not invariably result in a fall in blood pressure, and, moreover, when the pressure does fall, this may take several months.

Acute rises in blood pressure can be precipitated by interactions between tricyclic antidepressants and the adrenergic neurone-blocking drugs, guanethidine, bethanidine, and debrisoquine. The basis for this interaction depends on the property of the antidepressants to block the uptake of the hypotensive agent into the nerve ending, their site of action. Tricyclics also block the antihypertensive effect of clonidine, but not of α-methyldopa. A similar explanation can be given for the effect of proprietary cough and cold cures containing the indirectly acting amine phenylpropanolamine in reversing the antihypertensive effect of adrenergic neurone-blocking drugs. Better known, perhaps, is the potential of these cold cures to interact adversely with monoamine oxidase inhibitors, as do tyramine-containing foods and monoamine oxidase inhibitors. Sudden interruption of clonidine treatment can precipitate a considerable rise in blood pressure, and this can be accompanied by other manifestations of sympathetic overactivity such as tremor and tachycardia. These effects are exaggerated if the patient is taking a beta-adrenoceptor blocking drug that prevents only the beta (vasodilator) sympathetic response, leaving an unopposed alpha (vasoconstrictor) effect of the excess catecholamines. The remedy for the clonidine withdrawal syndrome is either rapid reintroduction of clonidine itself or administration of an alpha-adrenoceptor blocking agent, such as phentolamine.

Dangerous rises in blood pressure may also occur when patients are given vasopressor agents, such as noradrenaline and angiotensin, systematically. If noradrenaline were given to patients on tricyclic antidepressants an excessive rise in pressure might occur by virtue of the inhibition of neuronal uptake of the catecholamine. The response to noradrenaline is also exaggerated if the patient is on a drug such as guanethidine or reserpine, and this is caused by denervation hypersensitivity. Dopamine, a valuable agent in treating shock, increases renal blood flow and stimulates cardiac output in moderate doses. High doses can stimulate alpha-adrenoceptors and raise blood pressure considerably and may, incidentally, produce cardiac arrhythmias. Blood pressure must be monitored carefully when any vasopressor agent is being given.

DRUG-INDUCED HYPOTENSION

Hypotensive agents aside, several other unrelated drugs may lower blood pressure as an undesired effect. Among the best recorded are the phenothiazines, by virtue of their alpha-adrenoceptor blocking effect. This is especially important when this group of drugs are given with antihypertensive agents, and usually has a postural element. Many central depressant drugs will cause an unpredictable and unwanted fall in blood pressure, again often of a postural nature, and this may be more evident in the elderly.

PERIPHERAL ARTERIAL SPASM

Peripheral arterial spasm manifesting as Raynaud's phenomenon and occasionally progressing to gangrene has been seen in patients taking ergot-containing preparations to excess for migraine. Arterial spasm and occlusion also may occur when intravenous barbiturates or intravenous diazepam are injected intra-arterially in error.

THROMBOPHLEBITIS AND VENOUS THROMBOSIS

Local vein damage can occur as a result of any intravenous procedure —for instance, venepuncture or insertion of catheters—irrespective of any drug administered. Drugs most often implicated, however, are the antibiotics, amphotericin B and vancomycin, high-concentration sugar solutions, and, less often, diazepam. Considering the widespread use of intravenous contrast media and intravenous barbiturates, the overall risk of venous complications with them appears relatively small.

A major cuase for concern is venous thrombosis and thrombo-embolism with contraceptive steroids. The incidence of venous thrombosis is up to six times greater in women taking oral contraceptives, but with the increasing popularity of low-oestrogen-dose preparations the magnitude of this risk should decrease. Patients taking high doses of conjugated oestrogens also have an increased incidence of venous thrombosis, but when used in doses conventionally given for treating menopausal symptoms the risk is apparently not increased compared with a control population.

FURTHER READING

Davies, DM, ed. *Textbook of adverse drug reactions*. London: Oxford University Press, 1976.

Dukes, MNG, ed. *Meyler's side effects of drugs*. Vol 8. Amsterdam: Excerpta Medica, 1976.

Drug-induced neurological disease

E M R CRITCHLEY

Most clinicians acquire a wide practical knowledge of drug-induced disease. Drug trials and drug legislation cannot anticipate every circumstantial interaction or protoplasmic defect, and pharmaceutical research must continue to develop drugs, which of their nature cannot be subjected to large trials, to combat rare diseases. Patients and the public should respect the inevitability of side effects from powerful modern drugs, and doctors must improve their expertise in applied therapeutics and yet be prepared, where the possibility of adverse reactions arises, to seek the help of colleagues, hospital pharmacists, the Committee on Safety of Medicines, and medical representatives of the drug company concerned. The following discussion on drug-induced neurological disease is not intended to be comprehensive but rather to draw attention to some of the more important conditions.

Both old and young vary in their tolerance of drugs, and research is needed into the development of screening tests checking the patient's individual susceptibility to an iatrogenic challenge. For a few children the earliest challenge presented may arise from drugs that cross from the maternal to fetal circulation. Thus diazepam (Valium, Atensine) may cause respiratory depression in the newborn, lithium cause hypotonia, and antiemetics containing pyridoxine (for instance, Ancoloxin, Benadon, and Debendox) produce neonatal convulsions that require treatment with high doses of pyridoxine. Convulsions can also occur in breast-fed babies whose mothers are taking indomethacin (Indocid, Imbrilon). For most children the earliest risk of iatrogenic disease is that from vaccination, unmasking any constitutional weakness and given at a time of considerable susceptibility to intercurrent infection. The perils of pertussis vaccination are open to conflicting interpretations, however, and the relation to encephalopathy is far from proved.[2]

CEREBROSPINAL DISORDERS

All antibiotics are potentially neurotoxic. Given systemically the danger of convulsions and brain damage is potentiated by renal failure or blockade—as with probenecid (Colbenemid, Benemid), and this syndrome may also result from the intrathecal injection of noxious agents including undiluted penicillin or streptomycin. (No other antibiotic should be given by this route.) With high blood concentrations the aminoglycosides (streptomycin, kanamycin, and gentamicin) and the diuretics, ethacrynic acid (Edecrin), and frusemide (Lasix, Dryptal), are ototoxic. In contrast, aseptic meningitis may result from inadequate antibiotic treatment or poor penetration of the cerebrospinal fluid by wide-spectrum antibiotics. Bacterial meningitis and fungal disorders of the nervous system may arise during treatment with cytotoxic drugs or prolonged steroid administration. Another syndrome produced by drugs, including antibiotics, is iatrogenic intracranial hypertension (pseudotumour cerebri). The condition may present with bulging fontanelles, associated with the use of tetracycline in infancy, or arise in infants, children, teenagers, and young adults as a result of steroid administration (especially triamcinolone) or withdrawal, nalidixic acid (Negram), nitrofurantoin (Furadantin), or oral contraceptives.

CEREBROVASCULAR DISORDERS

Drugs affecting blood vessels and the constituents of the blood may all result in complications affecting the central nervous system. The incidence of complications from oral contraceptives has undoubtedly decreased since the introduction of the low oestrogen pill, but migraine may be intensified and drug-induced chorea, strokes, sinus thrombosis, subarachnoid haemorrhage, and subdural haematomas are still reported. Dexamethasone (Decadron), a powerful glucocorticoid, is invaluable in treating cerebral oedema, but its overenthusiastic use may result in failure to diagnose intracranial tumours or subdural haematomas. Other syndromes related to the administration of steroids include psychotic reactions, drug-sensitive relapsing polyneuritis, spinal compression from collapsed osteomalacic vertebrae, cataract, glaucoma, and a severe proximal myopathy that develops most readily when the fluorine-containing analogues are used but is seen with all steroid preparations.

MUSCULAR DISORDERS

Penicillamine, tetracycline, aminoglycosides—for instance, intraperitoneal streptomycin or neomycin—phenytoin, practolol, quinidine, and procainamide may compete with neuromuscular blocking agents and induce respiratory paralysis. Just occasionally, especially in the presence of renal failure, they may produce a true myasthenic syndrome, and anti-acetylcholine receptor antibodies have been identified in D-penicillamine-induced myasthenia gravis. Suxamethonium, alone or as the result of interaction with anaesthetic agents, can induce a syndrome of malignant hyperpyrexia and extreme muscular rigidity in genetically susceptible individuals. Drug-induced myopathies are caused by a wide variety of drugs including disulfiram, emetine, polymyxin E, allopurinol, and steroids. Many are improved on withdrawing treatment, thus aiding the differentiation from carcinomatous, endocrine, or metabolic myopathies.

PERIPHERAL NEUROPATHIES

Drugs may damage Schwann cells, myelin, axons, or the distal ends of peripheral nerves. Fibres of different sizes are selectively affected with manifestations affecting predominantly the motor or sensory nerves. Coexistent damage may affect anterior horn cells, cranial nerves, the eye, and muscles or other tissues of the body, so that, despite clinical variability, it is possible to distinguish distinctive patterns for particular drugs.

Isoniazid neuropathy is an axonal sensorimotor neuropathy with mental symptoms and skin changes similar to pellagra, and conditioned by a reversible pyridoxine depletion due to the genetically linked slow acetylation of isoniazid.

Thalidomide—Less notorious than phocomelia is the unpleasant burning dysaesthesiae of hands and feet with peripheral impairment of pain sensation often restricted to the digits after thalidomide. Unfortunately half of the patients remain without improvement after many years.

Nitrofurantoin (Furadantin) in the presence of renal impairment may, through failure of detoxication, lead to a refractory, symmetrical mixed neuropathy with reduced motor and sensory nerve conduction and segmental demyelination.

Clioquinol—A particularly virulent condition, subacute myelo-optic neuropathy, with a demyelinating syndrome of optic neuritis, myelopathy, and peripheral neuropathy has now been aetiologically linked with taking clioquinol (Enterovioform) for traveller's diarrhoea.

Chloroquine—With prolonged, high doses of chloroquine a motor polyneuropathy may develop. Recovery is rapid after drug withdrawal, but there may be an associated retinopathy and a myopathy with vacuolation and glycogen accumulation in muscle fibres.

Vinca alkaloids (vincristine and vinblastine), used to treat leukaemia, are particularly liable to neurotoxic effects, producing a painful sensorimotor polyneuropathy with axonal degeneration, secondary demyelination, and focal necrosis of muscle fibres. The autonomic nervous system may be involved, with constipation and intestinal obstruction, and, especially with intrathecal use, there may be extensive neuronal damage, convulsions, and ophthalmoplegia.

Perhexiline maleate (Pexid) may produce a reversible distal sensory neuropathy, proximal myopathy, and autonomic dysfunction with a raised protein content in cerebrospinal fluid that may lead to further complications.

Disopyramide (Norpace, Rhythmodan), another cardiac drug, may produce a mild sensorimotor neuropathy of larger fibre type with dysaesthesia of the feet.

Clofibrate (Atromid S) has occasionally produced a proximal myopathy with a distal motor neuropathy, severe myalgia, and muscle stiffness.

Drug-induced neurological disease

Disulfiram (*Antabuse*) and *cyanamide* (*Abstem*), used to treat alcohol addiction, can produce sensorimotor neuropathies and disulfiram may also cause optic neuritis and myopathy.

Metronidazole—A final example of a drug-induced polyneuropathy is that of metronidazole (Flagyl), used as a bactericide, protozoacide, and potentiating agent for radiotherapy. It may produce a mild distal sensory neuropathy, but occasionally a more severe neuritis with intolerable dysaesthesiae can result.

CONVULSIVE DISORDERS

The list of drugs capable of producing convulsions is formidable, and examples are given in order to emphasise how such reactions arise; from irritants injected into the subarachnoid space, such as penicillin, water-soluble contrast media, and antimitotic drugs; intravenous injections, particularly at an unstable pH—for instance, the penicillins and drugs to correct cardiac arrhythmias, such as lignocaine and disopyramide (Norpace, Rhythmodan); penetrative, antituberculosis drugs affecting pyridoxine metabolism, such as isoniazid and cycloserine; most antidepressives, including maprotiline (Ludiomil), amitryptiline (Tryptizol), and viloxazine (Vivalan), have mild cerebral irritant properties, and this function of chlorpromazine (Largactil) has been used to display instabilities in the electroencephalogram; hypoglycaemic agents, by causing too rapid a reduction in blood sugar; electrolyte imbalance, as from dilutional hyponatraemia caused by infusion of 5% dextrose water; and phenytoin in toxic doses becomes a convulsant, inducing attacks that may resemble hysteroepilepsy.

In narcotic institutions care is taken to titrate the withdrawal of barbiturates, more so than opiates, to prevent the risk to life of withdrawal fits. Similarly, if fits develop after a suicidal overdosage of barbiturates the treatment is always phenobarbitone and not other anticonvulsants. The cause of status epilepticus in established epilepsy is almost invariably the result of a reduction in anticonvulsants. Doctors should recognise that the taking of anticonvulsants is an imposition and that a psychological reaction is to be expected, particularly from teenagers. It is imperative to emphasise the advantages of regular medication in reducing the chances of kindling attacks in later life and to keep the regimen as simple and non-interfering as possible.

ANTICONVULSANT MEDICATION

Successful treatment with anticonvulsants depends on stable, therapeutic blood levels. Drug interactions, however, may occur in one or more phases of drug action: the drug release phase, for instance, within the intestine; the pharmacokinetic phase in which absorption, distribution, enzymic biotransformation, and excretion determine the concentration of the drug; and the pharmacodynamic phase in which drug and receptor combine to give a response.[1] Both phenobarbitone and phenytoin are potent inductors of hepatic enzymes lowering the serum concentrations of other drugs. At the same time, competition for plasma protein binding sites or inhibition of phenytoin metabolism by isoniazid or sulthiame (Ospolot) may rapidly produce toxic concentrations of phenytoin. The side effects of phenobarbitone include mental dulling and paradoxical hyperkinesia, especially when used in a brain-damaged child. Carbamazepine (Tegretol), an effective drug for focal epilepsy, may cause water intoxication and the practice of pushing fluids in a burnt epileptic child may thus be rendered hazardous.

However, the most commonly seen drug-induced neurological state without doubt is the subacute toxic-ataxic syndrome with anticonvulsants. Fine nystagmus occurs with therapeutic levels of phenytoin but coarse nystagmus, dysarthria, or ataxia is indicative of the toxic-ataxic syndrome. With variations—including hypotonia, truncal ataxia, drowsiness, and confusion—this syndrome is seen not only with phenytoin but with other anticonvulsants, such as primidone (Mysoline)—as an acute reaction on starting treatment—phenobarbitone, and carbamazepine (Tegretol). A less common syndrome and less readily diagnosed is the choreic-athetotic syndrome produced by toxic levels of the same drugs. The principal causes of these syndromes in practice are attempts to maintain patients on 400 mg or more of phenytoin without regular serum estimations or the thoughtless prescribing of combinations of Garoin (combined phenytoin and phenobarbitone) and phenytoin (Epanutin). Chronic phenytoin toxicity may lead to high levels of cerebrospinal fluid protein, encephalopathy, cerebellar degeneration, and a peripheral neuropathy (this latter is essentially of theoretical interest). Phenytoin is the best studied of all drugs and for this reason, perhaps, its side effects seem particularly horrendous. A myopathy has even been described as a sequel to anticonvulsant osteomalacia.

EXTRAPYRAMIDAL AND ALLIED SYNDROMES

Few non-psychiatrists have the opportunity to study the normal responses of patients to lithium carbonate (Camcolit, Phasal, Priadel). Lithium salts are prescribed to treat and prevent manic-depressive episodes and probably act by altering electrolyte and amine levels in the brain. The toxic effects may include bizarre combinations of neurological symptoms, which are inadequately described in published reports; thus, to quote a personal case, I was asked whether a patient who happened to be taking lithium had Parkinsonism, cerebrovascular disease, or an underlying tumour. He appeared depressed with a slow, thick hesitant speech, kept one eye closed because of photophobia, had bilateral hand tremor, ankle clonus, flexor plantar responses, and locomotor apraxia. He responded dramatically to a reduction in the dose of lithium carbonate.

The side effects that may occur with plasma concentrations below 1·8 mmol/l include fine tremor, weakness, polydipsia, polyuria, hypothyroidism, and hypokalaemia; and any disturbance of water or electrolyte balance—as from diuretics, strict dieting, and sauna baths or interaction with potentially nephrotoxic agents such as tetracycline—can precipitate more serious reactions. Within the lower toxic range these may include ataxia, blurred vision, confusion, drowsiness, fasciculation, and slurred speech; and, with more severe poisoning, hyperreflexia, entensor spasms, convulsions, toxic psychosis, syncope, and coma. Serious interactions can occur with haloperidol, phenytoin, and diazepam. Lithium potentiates the side effects of other psychotropic drugs but combined treatment is possible, provided such drugs are started at a lower dosage than usual.

All effective major tranquillisers are capable of inducing extrapyramidal disturbances. This propensity is seen mainly with the piperazine series of phenothiazines (Stelazine, Stemetil, Fentazin, and fluphenazine), and butyrophenones (haloperidol); but a mild Parkinsonian syndrome can also occur in older patients on tricyclic antidepressants and with reserpine or tetrabenazine (Nitoman). Extrapyramidal movement disorders may follow the withdrawal of antihistamines, glutethimide (Doriden), antidepressants, and narcotics, probably due to an imbalance between cholinergic and dopaminergic activity in the basal ganglia, or be induced by the antimalarial amodiaquine (Camoquin). In one series[3] 40% of patients treated for major psychoses with phenothiazines developed extrapyramidal reactions: about 21% developed akathiasis (motor restlessness), 16% Parkinsonism, and 3% dystonias—torticollis, writhing, grimacing, and oculogyric crises. These dose-related disorders are usually reversible; but not so the persistent (tardive) dyskinesias, which are related to the total amount ingested. Tardive dyskinesias are the scourge of long-stay mental institutions, affecting 12% of male and 20% of female patients.[4] Typically, they affect the bucco-linguo-masticatory muscles in quasi-compulsive, stereotyped movements that may simulate the potentially reversible dyskinetic movements produced by levodopa. There is no value in the prophylactic administration of anticholinergic drugs for these conditions, and drug-induced Parkinsonism does not respond to levodopa. Retinal damage may result from the piperidine derivatives such as thioridazine (Melleril); and haloperidol (Seranace) has proved unsafe in thyrotoxicosis. A particular warning[1] is given against using the antiemetic metoclopramide (Maxolon) in childhood, as a single dose may incite acute dystonia or a reaction simulating an acute encephalopathy.

The incidence of severe side effects with monoamine oxidase inhibitors is highest in patients who are slow acetylators of isoniazid. Acute reactions include insomnia, agitation, hallucinations, hyperreflexia, hyperpyrexia with neck rigidity, convulsions, and hypo- or hyper-tension. More chronic side effects include tremor, peripheral neuropathy, orthostatic hypotension, hypomania, oculomotor paralysis, and toxic amblyopia; but most hazardous are the hypertensive reactions with headache and intracranial haemorrhage when a monoamine oxidase inhibitor is given simultaneously with certain drugs or foods. The adverse neurological manifestations of the tricyclic antidepressants and allied drugs usually stem from their anticholinergic actions, precipitating glaucoma, convulsions, or various states of hallucinosis, delirium, or manic excitement. With acute overdosage, hyperpyrexia, hypertension, and seizures may result in a coma potentially reversible with physostigmine. The major hazard of the benzodiazepines comes from the variability of response: thus a paradoxical reaction can occur with excitement or depression instead of sedation. There is also the risk of dependence of the barbiturate-alcohol type with withdrawal reactions including convulsions and potentiation of other drugs; thus hypotonia, ataxia, erratic behaviour, and drowsiness may be observed with clonazepam (Rivotril), especially when used in conjunction with other anticonvulsants.

Parkinsonism is a degenerative disease often accompanied by depression and loss of drug tolerance. Although anticholinergic drugs may add to the risk of confusional states, they act synergistically with levodopa and their subsequent withdrawal may lead to hypersalivation and intense rigidity. Currently, an immediate problem is the need to nullify the dyskinetic and on-off effects resulting from long-term treatment with levodopa. In this regard the efficacy of bromocriptine (used successfully in lower dosage of endocrine dysfunction, anorexia nervosa, and hypertension) has been questioned. Twenty-five to 40% of Parkinsonian patients are unable to tolerate therapeutic doses of this drug, and in those who have received levodopa refractory visual hallucinations and confusional states often occur.[5] Bromocriptine may also have the harmful effect of hypersensitising dopaminergic receptors.[6]

The most serious omissions in this review include a description of drugs that produce confusional states, depression, or damage the ocular system. Drug syndromes should always be considered, especially when a patient apparently benefiting from treatment suddenly develops untoward and unexplained symptoms.

REFERENCES

[1] *British National Formulary*, 1976–8. Aylesbury: Hazell, Watson and Viney.

[2] Miller DL, Ross EM. National childhood encephalopathy study: an interim report. *Br Med J* 1978;ii:992–3.

[3] Ayd FJ. A survey of drug induced extrapyramidal reactions. *JAMA* 1961;**175**:1054–60.
[4] Lader MH. Drug induced extrapyramidal syndromes. *J R Coll Physicians London* 1970;**5**:87–98.
[5] Stern G, Lees A. Bromocriptine in Parkinson's disease. *Br J Hosp Med* 1978;**206**:666–70.
[6] Nausieda PA, Weiner WJ, Kanapa DJ, Klawans HL. Bromocriptine-induced behavioural hypersensitivity: implications for the therapy of Parkinsonism. *Neurology* 1978;**28**:1183–8.

Drug-induced skin diseases

R A HARDIE, J A SAVIN

Drug eruptions are a bit like the Joneses: no one ever quite seems able to keep up with them. The problem is that as soon as the older drugs slip out of use, taking with them their familiar rashes, new fashionable treatments are rushed out of the laboratories. It is often a long time before any one can accept that they also will cause trouble. Practolol was a good example of this: used widely since 1970, it was not until 1974 that its now well-known skin reactions were described.[1]

In other ways, however, though drugs may change, the clinical problems remain depressingly the same: a patient develops a rash; he is taking many different tablets; which, if any, of these caused his eruption, and what should be done about it? It is no answer simply to stop all drugs, though the fact that this can often be done casts some doubt on the patient's need for them in the first place. All too often potentially valuable drugs are excluded from further use on totally inadequate grounds. Clearly some guidelines are needed, but no simple set of rules exists that can cover this complex subject. In this short article we can do no more than outline some commonsense steps in the approach to patients with possible drug-induced skin disease. We suggest that the following questions should be asked in every case: (1) Can other skin diseases be excluded? (2) Are the skin changes compatible with a drug cause? (3) Which drug is most likely to be responsible? (4) Are any further tests worth while? and (5) Is any treatment needed? These questions are deceptively simple but the answers are often difficult. Each step will be discussed in turn.

CAN OTHER SKIN DISEASES BE EXCLUDED?

The fact that a patient is taking tablets does not mean that he cannot suffer from one of the ordinary dermatoses. Scabies, psoriasis, or eczema, which the patient may have had for a long time, may first be noted by a sharp-eyed houseman in the ward, and be thought to be a drug eruption. Perhaps the commonest condition that is mistaken for a drug eruption is asteatotic eczema. This often starts after admission to a ward but is due to fierce washing by the nursing staff rather than to drugs, and the use of diuretics may be a predisposing factor. A highly itchy rash is seen on the already dry skin, usually of the legs, of elderly patients, and can be recognised by its pink linear splits in the stratum corneum.

Occasionally, of course, skin conditions are made worse by drugs given for other diseases. For example, antimalarials (especially chloroquine and mepacrine) and lithium may worsen psoriasis. Acne and dermatitis herpetiformis may flare up after taking cough mixtures containing iodides. Acne can also be induced or made worse by corticosteroids (given after puberty), testosterone, phenobarbitone, phenytoin, and INAH. Oral contraceptives with a high progesterone content are best avoided by women with a tendency to develop acne.

ARE THE SKIN CHANGES COMPATIBLE WITH A DRUG CAUSE?

Almost every medical journal contains at least one description of a drug-induced skin disorder, and the thick fall of papers has tended to obscure the outlines of the subject. The same drug may produce completely different eruptions in different patients and quite unrelated drugs may cause similar eruptions. There are, however, several set patterns of reaction that are often drug induced. A thumbnail sketch of some of the commonest ones is given below.

Toxic erythema is the commonest skin reaction to drugs, and the term is used to describe many patterns of erythema. Sometimes the lesions look like measles, or scarlet fever; sometimes an urticarial or erythema-multiforme-like element is prominent; and the lesions may be macular or papular. The lesions are often more pronounced on the trunk than on the extremities. In previously exposed patients the rash may start two to three days after the administration of a drug. If a reaction arises during the first course of treatment the eruption will take longer to develop, often appearing about the ninth day. Fever may accompany the skin reaction. Unfortunately the drug that is responsible cannot usually be identified from the appearance of the rash. Common culprits include antibiotics (especially ampicillin), sulphonamides and related compounds (including thiazide diuretics, frusemide, and sulphonylurea hypoglycaemics), barbiturates, phenylbutazone, and para-aminosalicylic acid.

Erythema multiforme—The target-like lesions appear mainly on the extensor aspect of the limbs. In severe cases bullae may form. Occasionally the mucous membranes are severely affected (the Stevens-Johnson syndrome). Sulphonamides, barbiturates, and phenylbutazone are the commonest offenders.

Erythema nodosum—Sulphonamides and the oral contraceptive pill may produce this well-known reaction pattern.

Allergic vasculitis—In this reaction the inflammatory changes are most severe round blood vessels, especially veins and venules. The clinical changes range from urticaria to necrotic ulcers, and many confusing variants have been described. The sulphonamides, phenylbutazone, indomethacin, and phenytoin, are possible causes.

Purpura—Drugs may produce purpura by causing thrombocytopenia, by damaging the blood vessel, or by affecting blood coagulation. The clinical features of drug purpura are seldom distinctive apart from the itchy, brownish, petechial rash on dependent areas that is characteristic of carbromal reactions. Thiazides, sulphonamides, phenylbutazone, sulphonylureas, barbiturates, and quinine are among the drugs reported to cause purpura.

Eczema is a rare result of drug treatment and is characterised by a predominantly epidermal reaction similar to contact dermatitis. It is usually seen when patients, previously sensitised by external exposure, are given the same or a related substance systemically. Penicillin, neomycin, the phenothiazines, and local anaesthetics are common examples.

Exfoliative dermatitis and erythrodermia are descriptive terms used when the entire skin surface is red and scaly. An identical appearance is produced by drugs (phenylbutazone, para-aminosalicylic acid, isoniazid, gold, carbamazepine), severe psoriasis or eczema, or a lymphoma.

Photosensitivity may be defined as an exaggerated response of the skin to ultraviolet light. The rash typically affects the exposed skin of the face, neck, and backs of the hands, and also, in women, the lower legs. Both phototoxic and photoallergic mechanisms may be responsible, but in practice the distinction is often difficult to make. Exacerbations are usually related to spells of good weather, but on occasion the ultraviolet emission from fluorescent lighting may be sufficient. The most common photosensitisers are sulphonamides, sulphonamide-related compounds (thiazide diuretics, frusemide, and sulphonylurea hypoglycaemics), tetracyclines (especially demethylchlortetracycline), phenothiazines, and nalidixic acid.

Drug-related lupus erythematosus may present with a photosensitive rash accompanied by fever, polyarthritis, myalgia, and serositis (pleural and pericardial). The antinuclear factor is invariably present, but antibodies to double-stranded DNA are absent. The illness tends to be less severe than systemic lupus erythematosus and complete recovery often follows withdrawal of the drug, although antinuclear factor may be present for some time. Hydrallazine, isoniazid, procainamide, and phenytoin are the commonest causes, but many drugs have been incriminated.

Lichenoid eruptions is a term used to describe eruptions resembling lichen planus. In addition to the flat-topped papules there is often scaling and dermatitic change. The mouth is seldom affected. Chloroquine, mepacrine, gold, arsenic, phenothiazines, and para-aminosalicylic acid are some of the drugs known to cause this reaction.

Fixed eruptions consist of demarcated, round, erythematous plaques that characteristically recur at the same site each time the drug is given. Persistent pigmentation remains after healing. Phenolphthalein, barbiturates, sulphonamides, quinine, and tetracycline may be responsible.

Toxic epidermal necrolysis—In rare cases large sheets of erythema develop and are followed by separation of the epidermis, giving the appearance of scalded skin. Staphylococcal infection (phage type 71) is usually responsible in infants, but in adults the eruption has followed treatment with barbiturates, phenytoin, sulphonamides, phenylbutazone, oxyphenbutazone, and penicillin.

Urticaria—Drugs are rarely the cause of chronic urticaria, but the penicillins and salicylates may be responsible especially in atopic individuals. Aspirin also acts as a non-specific histamine-releasing agent, and patients with urticaria should therefore avoid it. Enough penicillin may be present in dairy products to cause chronic urticaria in penicillin-sensitive patients.

Pruritus—An itchy skin not associated with a rash may be the only evidence of a drug reaction. The contraceptive pill, phenothiazines, and rifampicin may produce this symptom due to biliary stasis. Pruritus ani may be caused by the overgrowth of candida after systemic antibiotic treatment.

Hair loss is a predictable side effect of drugs such as cytotoxic agents and oral contraceptives. Diffuse hair loss also occurs unpredictably with anticoagulants (heparin, coumarins, and phenindione) and antithyroid drugs (carbimazole and thiouracil).

Pigmentation—Drugs can cause many different types of pigmentary upset. Perhaps the most common is the development of flat, hyperpigmented areas on the forehead and cheeks (chloasma) caused by oral contraceptives; unfortunately this pigmentation is slow to improve despite stopping the drug. Chlorpromazine and related phenothiazines cause a blue-grey discoloration on light-exposed areas. Heavy metals (silver, gold, bismuth, and arsenic) produce a generalised brown or blue-grey pigmentation. A uniform yellow colour may result from mepacrine treatment, while chloroquine produces blue-black patches on the shins, pigmentation of the nails and palate, and depigmentation of the hair.

WHICH DRUG IS MOST LIKELY TO BE RESPONSIBLE?

The patient is still there, liberally dappled with his rash; ordinary dermatoses have been excluded; and the clinical pattern of the rash has been identified as compatible with a drug reaction. Now the problem is to decide which of his many drugs has been responsible for the eruption. Very few drugs are so obliging as to cause an eruption that is absolutely specific; indeed, most drugs can, at one time or another, cause most types of drug rash, though some tend to give rise to particular rashes more often than others.

A knowledge of each drug's track record is all important, and for those without wide personal experience, the best policy is to consult published reports. Bruinsma's *A Guide to Drug Eruptions*[2] remains a useful dogmatic guide. The known behaviour of individual drugs can best be found in standard text books.[3 4]

Further help may come from a look at the dates on the prescription sheets. It is quite true that a drug taken for years may suddenly cause a reaction, but this is rather less common than an eruption appearing only a few days after a drug has been started. From this it would seem that the drug most recently introduced into a treatment regimen may be the most likely culprit. But often the records show a bewildering succession of drugs, sometimes in twos or threes, given in brief bursts during a protracted illness. Even a dermatologist cannot always sort out this sort of a mess.

Once the offending drug has been stopped, the eruption will usually start to improve within a few days, though some types, such as lichenoid eruptions, may clear much more slowly. Continued exposure to the substance in an unexpected form (for instance, penicillin in milk) may confuse the issue.

ARE ANY FURTHER TESTS WORTHWHILE?

In-vivo tests

Readministration—With the possible exception of a fixed eruption, readministration is hazardous. It may produce anaphylactic shock with death in a few minutes. The results can also be misleading as the test dose used should be small and hence may be too small to elicit a reaction. Readministration is probably justified only when no suitable alternative drug exists, and where hyposensitisation might be attempted. One exception is the rash so often seen after ampicillin has been given to patients with glandular fever. Once the mononucleosis has cleared ampicillin can usually be given again with impunity.

Patch tests only detect delayed type hypersensitivity and are therefore of limited use except in contact allergy and perhaps the rare eczematous type of drug eruption. Patch tests may be positive on the plaque of a fixed drug eruption though negative on the rest of the skin.

Prick and scratch tests introduce a small amount of the allergen into the dermis. The preparation of the allergen is of the utmost importance since most drugs act only as allergens after combining with a protein or other macromolecule. In most cases, unfortunately, we do not know how to prepare the complete allergen. Even with penicillin, where a considerable amount is known about the allergic determinants, a negative reaction to the major haptenic determinant (using penicilloyl-polylysine) does not mean the patient will not react adversely to untested minor determinants when given the drug. These procedures may also produce anaphylaxis and may even induce allergy. The actual injection of small quantities into the dermis is perhaps more reliable than prick or scratch testing but carries a higher risk of anaphylaxis. The reservations expressed above about testing to the correct allergen apply equally to intradermal injections.

In-vitro tests

In-vitro tests are useful only in drug reactions of allergic origin. It must be emphasised that the detection of drug-specific circulating antibodies proves only the occurrence of an immunological response to that particular drug, and not that the clinical reaction was due to it. Tests for immediate-type drug allergy (anaphylaxis) include detection of reaginic antibodies, measurement of allergen-specific IgE antibodies (RAST), the basophil degranulation test, and the red-cell-linked antigen-antiglobulin reaction (RCLAAR). Type II reactions have been investigated using the direct and indirect antiglobulin tests (Coombs test), inhibition of clot retraction, complement fixation tests, and mixed antiglobulin reactions. Evidence of type III reactions includes measurement of circulating immune complexes (for instance, Clq precipitation) and the demonstration of antigen-antibody-complement complexes in tissues by immunofluorescence. Methods for detecting delayed type hypersensitivity (type IV) are the lymphocyte transformation test and the macrophage migration inhibition test.

The laboratory methods listed above are still largely experimental and do not yield consistent results. In addition they require facilities that are not usually available to the clinician.

IS ANY TREATMENT NEEDED?

The first approach to treatment of a suspected adverse drug reaction is to withdraw the drug, but several drugs may have to be stopped to ensure that this is done, since it may be impossible to pinpoint the culprit.

Anaphylactic reactions occur so rapidly that the patient presents as an acute medical emergency. Adrenaline is the most effective treatment, and 0.5 ml of 1 in 1000 solution should be injected subcutaneously and repeated if necessary after five minutes. An antihistamine (such as chlorpheniramine maleate 20 mg) should also be administered parenterally as soon as possible. Corticosteroids are of limited use in the acute phase, but hydrocortisone hemisuccinate, 100–300 mg, given intramuscularly soon after the onset may prove beneficial later.

Most adverse drug reactions, however, are much less dramatic and will subside in a few days after the drug is stopped. Only symptomatic treatment is required with topical calamine lotion or crotamiton (Eurax) lotion and a systemic antihistamine—for instance, trimeprazine 10 mg thrice daily. If the reaction is severe a tapering course of oral prednisolone is sometimes given—for example, in the Stevens-Johnson syndrome—but often there is not much objective evidence that this treatment speeds up resolution.

CONCLUSION

This whole subject is shot through with uncertainties. Even the incidence of drug eruptions seems to be hard to estimate. Most authors reckon that between 1 and 5% of all patients in hospital will develop a drug eruption of one kind or another, and this incidence is inexcusably high.

What can be done about this? Prevention would be better than cure, and the more rigorous screening and purification of drugs before general release might help here. There is, however, still much to be done by the clinician. No one who is asked to see drug eruptions regularly can fail to be depressed by the vast flickering sequence of drugs to which many patients are exposed. Every symptom does not always need drug treatment, and the national drug bills as well as the incidence of drug eruptions could be slashed if all doctors declared war on polypharmacy. Failing this, the laborious and often unsatisfactory clinical detective work must continue, based on probabilities and common sense, and largely unaided by complicated and unreliable laboratory tests.

REFERENCES

[1] Felix RH, Ive FA, Dahl MGC. Cutaneous and ocular reations to practolol. *Br Med J* 1974;iv:321–4.
[2] Bruinsma W. *A guide to drug eruptions*. Amsterdam; Excerpta Medica, 1973.
[3] Martindale. In: Blacow NW, ed. *The extra pharmacopoeia*. London: Pharmaceutical Press, 1972.
[4] Baker H. In: Rook A, Wilkinson DS, Ebling FJG, eds. *Textbook of dermatology*. London: Blackwell, 1972:chap 35.

Drug-induced respiratory disease

I W B GRANT

It has been common knowledge for many years that some drugs in everyday use may cause or aggravate respiratory disease. Familiar examples are aspirin, which can provoke an acute attack of asthma; opiates and barbiturates, which can precipitate ventilatory failure in chronic bronchitis; and liquid paraffin, which can spill over from the oesophagus into the trachea and produce lipoid pneumonia. Nevertheless, it was not until recently that the concept of drug-induced respiratory disease engaged the attention and interest of the medical profession. Although the bronchi and lungs are less vulnerable to the harmful effects of drugs than the gastrointestinal tract, liver, kidneys, and nervous system, reported instances of drug-induced respiratory disease have steadily increased. This must be due in part to the introduction of new therapeutic agents, but other factors may include a higher index of suspicion that any obscure respiratory illness may be drug-induced and an increasing awareness that the administration of therapeutic agents, such as antibiotics and immunosuppressive drugs, which have no specific action on the lungs, may indirectly be responsible for pulmonary disease, particularly infections.

Drugs can affect the respiratory system by:

(1) exerting specific pharmacological effects on bronchial calibre or pulmonary function;

(2) mediating allergic reactions in the bronchi or lungs;

(3) inducing a syndrome resembling systemic lupus erythematosus with pulmonary and pleural manifestations;

(4) producing various obscure forms of diffuse pulmonary disease affecting the alveoli or the alveolar walls or both;

(5) exposing patients to opportunist pulmonary infections with bacteria, viruses, fungi, or protozoa as a consequence of therapeutic immunosuppression or broad-spectrum antibacterial therapy;

(6) disturbing the normal mechanisms of coagulation and causing either thromboembolic disease or pulmonary haemorrhage; and

(7) producing focal lesions in the lungs when inhaled accidentally or a diagnostic or therapeutic measure.

SPECIFIC PHARMACOLOGICAL EFFECTS

Opiates, barbiturates, and even milder sedative drugs, such as nitrazepam or diazepam, cause central depression of respiration and may be responsible for the onset of ventilatory failure in patients with chronic airflow obstruction (bronchitis and emphysema) and bronchial asthma. Oxygen treatment, by reducing hypoxic respiratory drive in these subjects, may have the same effect if the inspired oxygen concentration is too high.

In a different category are drugs used in treating various non-respiratory disorders, which cause bronchoconstriction either by parasympathetic stimulation (cholinergic drugs) or by beta-adrenoreceptor blockade. The most commonly prescribed drugs in the second category are propranolol and oxprenolol, both of which may provoke severe bronchospasm in patients with asthma. The newer "cardio-selective" beta-blocking drugs, such as metoprolol, acebutolol, and atenolol, although less apt to induce bronchoconstriction, may do so in some asthmatic patients, and should be prescribed with equal caution in such individuals.

ALLERGIC REACTIONS

Allergic rhinitis, bronchial asthma, and pulmonary eosinophilia may result from taking a variety of therapeutic agents. These include proteins with inherent antigenic potential, such as antisera and vaccines, and certain drugs of low molecular weight acting as haptens (substances that acquire antigenic properties when chemically bound to a protein). In sensitised individuals, all these therapeutic agents can produce or aggravate allergic respiratory disease, but there is considerable variation both between drugs and between patients in the nature of their clinical effects. In some cases there may be rhinitis or asthma, either alone or in combination. In others, pulmonary eosinophilia may occur as an isolated phenomenon, or may be accompanied by bronchial asthma. Extrinsic allergic alveolitis seems to be an uncommon manifestation of drug-induced respiratory disease. The drugs reported to cause these various forms of allergic reaction are listed in table 1.

Aspirin provokes acute bronchoconstriction in asthmatic patients more often than any other drug, possibly because it is consumed at one time or another by almost every member of the population. A similar asthmatic reaction may, however, follow the administration of other analgesic and anti-inflammatory drugs, such as paracetamol, phenylbutazone, and indomethacin, and of tartrazine, an orange-yellow azo dye used to colour many commonly prescribed drugs. Most of these substances, including aspirin, are known to inhibit prostaglandin synthesis, and that is believed to increase the release of slow reacting substance of anaphylaxis (SRS-A), a powerful bronchoconstrictor, from mast cells in the bronchi. Not all asthmatic patients are aspirin-sensitive, but those who are must be warned never to take that drug again, and their doctors must exercise caution in prescribing other analgesics or any orange-yellow-coloured tablets. A hazard which such patients should be taught to recognise and avoid is that aspirin is a constituent of many of the patent pain-killing tablets which are on sale to the public.

Sensitivity to aspirin may not have an immunological basis, and the same may be true of sensitivity to iodine. Reactions to iodine-containing contrast media used in radiology may take the form of acute anaphylaxis, with severe bronchoconstriction. This is probably due to a massive release of histamine caused by direct action of these substances on mast cells. That is unlikely to be mediated by an antigen-antibody reaction since it can occur in patients who have never before been investigated with iodine-containing contrast media. "Iodism" is a milder and more chronic form of sensitivity to iodine, usually when given as a cough mixture containing potassium iodide, and its most common respiratory manifestation is bronchorrhoea.

PULMONARY AND PLEURAL MANIFESTATIONS OF A DRUG-INDUCED SYNDROME RESEMBLING SYSTEMIC LUPUS ERYTHEMATOSUS

Some drugs, including hydrallazine, procainamide, practolol, isoniazid, and phenytoin, are known to give rise to a syndrome closely resembling systemic lupus erythematosus, both clinically and serologically. These patients often develop diffuse pulmonary lesions and pleural thickening.

Patients usually recover when the drug is withdrawn, but the observation that in some instances the condition persists, and even progresses, raises the question as to whether the action of these drugs is merely to uncover latent forms of the disease.

TABLE I—*Drugs reported to cause allergic respiratory disorders*

Bronchial asthma	Penicillin and other antibiotics Antisera and vaccines Allergenic extracts used for hyposensitisation Aspirin Monoamine-oxidase inhibitors Iodine-containing contrast media Iron dextran
Bronchorrhoea	Iodides
Pulmonary eosinophilia	Nitrofurantoin Para-aminosalicylic acid Sulphasalazine Other sulphonamides Imipramine Chlorpropamide Phenylbutazone Aspirin Penicillin and other antibiotics
Allergic alveolitis	Pituitary snuff

OTHER TYPES OF DIFFUSE PULMONARY DISEASE

Drug-induced lung disease in this category is not associated with identifiable immune responses, and it has been postulated that they may be related to some form of enzymatic abnormality. They form a heterogeneous histopathological group, ranging from the desquamative alveolitis and interstitial fibrosis caused by the cytotoxic drugs busulphan and bleomycin to a syndrome resembling adult hyaline membrane disease ("fibrinous pneumonia"), which has been observed after treatment with the now obsolete antihypertensive drug methonium and some related compounds, and to overdosage of the tricyclic antidepressive amitriptyline.

The pathological changes in the second group bear some resemblance to those seen in pulmonary oxygen toxicity (itself to be regarded as a form of drug-induced lung disease) and paraquat poisoning. It is conceivable that these conditions may all be related to inhibition of surfactant production in the pulmonary alveoli.

OPPORTUNIST PULMONARY INFECTIONS

With the increasing use of cytotoxic drugs in malignant disease, immunosuppressive drugs in transplantation surgery and in the treatment of diseases such as bronchial asthma and autoimmune disorders, and of broad-spectrum antibiotic treatment, many patients are now being exposed to the risk of developing opportunist pulmonary infection (table II). Although these infections might not be regarded as specific

TABLE II—*Examples of drug-induced opportunist pulmonary infections*

Bacterial	*Staphylococcus pyogenes* Gram-negative bacilli *Mycobacterium tuberculosis*
Viral	Cytomegalovirus
Fungal	*Aspergillus fumigatus* *Candida albicans* *Cryptococcus neoformans*
Protozoal	*Pneumocystis carinii*

forms of drug-induced lung disease, they are numerically important, and probably account for more fatalities than all the other drugs discussed in this article.

It is clearly essential to make a positive microbiological diagnosis in these cases at the earliest possible stage, so that treatment can be started without delay. The technique of transbronchial lung biopsy may be required in cases of suspected *Pneumocystis carinii* pneumonia.

Drug-induced respiratory disease

COAGULATION DISORDERS CAUSING PULMONARY THROMBOEMBOLISM OR PULMONARY HAEMORRHAGE

Oestrogen-containing oral contraceptives predispose to pulmonary thromboembolism, but even with the aid of modern investigative procedures it is often extremely difficult to determine whether or not an episode of pleural pain is due to pulmonary infection, and to decide if the contraceptive pill should be withdrawn. Cytotoxic drugs may cause haemoptysis by reducing the platelet count.

FOCAL PULMONARY LESIONS CAUSED BY INHALATION

Nasal drops or sprays consisting of vasoconstrictive drugs suspended in liquid paraffin were once a not uncommon cause of lipoid granulomas in the lungs, but those forms of treatment have now been abandoned. This type of lesion is, however, still seen occasionally in patients who consume large amounts of liquid paraffin for constipation, because small quantities of this mineral oil may ooze into the trachea during swallowing.

Much larger quantities may enter the air passages in patients with cardiospasm, who often have an incompetent cricopharyngeal sphincter, and such patients may develop extensive lipoid pneumonia. Iodine-containing opaque media suspended in arachis oil, used for bronchographic examination, may also produce lipoid granulomas.

CONCLUSION

There are two main reasons why doctors are often slow to recognise drug-induced respiratory disease. The first is failure to elicit detailed information about patients' current or recent drug treatment. The second is ignorance of the identity of those therapeutic agents that are capable of producing bronchial and pulmonary disease. It may also be the case that recently introduced drugs, not mentioned in this article, may prove to have adverse effects, so far unrecognised, on the respiratory system, and the vital importance of reporting every suspected case of drug-induced disease to the Committee on Safety of Medicines cannot be over-emphasised.

Drug-induced metabolic disease

P RICHARDS

All drug-induced disease is metabolic; this chapter is confined to drug-induced disturbances of water and electrolyte, urate, and carbohydrate metabolism. To avoid pitfalls in common conditions is its prime purpose. No attempt is made to present a comprehensive review of drug-induced metabolic disease, or to explore the mechanisms of such disease in any detail. The points touched on here are mostly common knowledge, but failure to apply this knowledge is, unfortunately, also common.

WATER AND ELECTROLYTE METABOLISM

Salt and water retention

Patients with incipient heart failure or oedema from any cause are at risk from the following common drugs: anti-inflammatory drugs such as phenylbutazone and indomethacin; carbenoxolone; tricyclic antidepressants; oestrogens; and hypotensive drugs. All these promote salt and water retention. Hypotensive drugs have a non-specific homoeostatic salt and water retaining effect proportional to the fall in blood pressure and some also have additional mechanisms—for example, potent vasodilators such as diazoxide and minoxidil are intensely salt-retaining out of proportion to the fall in blood pressure; beta-adrenoceptor blockers predispose to oedema partly on account of a negative inotropic effect on the heart.

Excessive intravenous infusion of sodium is a commonly overlooked cause of saline overload on both medical and surgical wards, largely from failure to consider intake in relation to the variable ability to excrete salt and water during illness or after surgical operation. Problems should be few if the patient is carefully examined daily (especially for oedema); is weighed daily; and if only a few simple intravenous solutions are used so that intake can readily be calculated. Intravenous fluids must be prescribed with deliberation and care, and only one day at a time—sometimes less. It is important not to give intravenous nutrition without considering the fluid and electrolyte consequences: some amino-acid solutions, for example, contain 120–150 mmol (mEq) of sodium per litre, enough by itself for most patients and too much for those whose renal function is still under the shadow of operation.

Salt and water depletion

Even with great care it is difficult to avoid sometimes making patients ill with diuretics. The usual cause is failure to reduce the dose of diuretic soon after the onset of a satisfactory diuresis; normally a diuresis is more difficult to induce than to maintain; and it is usually both possible and desirable to reduce the dose during treatment.

Diuretic treatment should always be reviewed periodically to ensure that the dose is appropriate (especially when other strongly protein-bound drugs are given that increase the plasma concentration of free diuretic by displacement) and indeed that the treatment is still necessary at all. An excessively large or rapid diuresis may profoundly reduce cardiac output, especially in the elderly, causing weakness, confusion, and deteriorating renal function.

Hyponatraemia and hypernatraemia

The plasma sodium concentration indicates the balance between salt and water—by itself, it gives no certain information about overall saline deficiency or excess. If thirst and antidiuretic hormone (ADH) release are normal they together ensure that saline retention or loss is isotonic and that the plasma sodium concentration therefore is in the normal range. Drug-induced hyponatraemia has two causes: replacement of salt loss (commonly diuretic-induced) with water, and an ADH-like action of drugs (such as chlorpropamide and carbamazepine). Further complexity occurs in serious disease because of the associated inappropriate secretion of ADH. The implicated drug must be stopped and water restricted (sometimes to as little as 500 ml daily at first); in emergency, slow intravenous infusion of up to 250 ml of five-times physiological saline (4·5 g/l) is indicated but it carries a risk of acute heart failure in predisposed patients; it is neither necessary nor wise to attempt rapidly to correct the plasma sodium fully to normal.

Hypernatraemia almost invariably indicates water depletion, combined sometimes with excessive sodium intake as, for example, when unconscious patients are tube-fed with hypertonic solutions containing a large amount of both sodium and protein. More salt is supplied than water, and urea derived from the protein induces an osmotic urea diuresis, adding an absolute water deficiency to the previous relative deficiency; hypertonic feeds also cause diarrhoea with further loss of water. Similar risks, without the diarrhoea, exist with intravenous feeding: rapid hypertonic glucose infusion may exceed glucose tolerance causing glycosuria with osmotic diuresis; amino-acids are converted to urea causing urea diuresis; and many solutions add sodium to the insult of osmotic water loss. Over-diuresis of patients unable to respond to thirst because of impaired consciousness is another iatrogenic cause of hypernatraemia.

Hypokalaemia and hyperkalaemia

Drug-induced hypokalaemia is usually attributable to diuretics, adrenal corticosteroids, or carbenoxolone (which has a mineralocorticoid-like action on the distal tubule). Small potassium supplements do not reliably prevent hypokalaemia in patients taking thiazides or loop diuretics nor are they routinely necessary, but the elderly and patients taking digoxin should receive a supplement sufficient to maintain a normal plasma potassium concentration. The plasma concentration must be checked at least once at about three months because requirements vary considerably, and no standard dose (whether in a combined tablet of diuretic and potassium or not) can be relied on to be sufficient. Hypokalaemia is best prevented in patients with chronic heart failure or hypoproteinaemic oedema who are taking thiazides or loop diuretics by simultaneous treatment with spironolactone, which competitively inhibits secondary hyperaldosteronism. Most other patients taking thiazides (the most appropriate diuretics for treating hypertension) do not need a routine potassium supplement; measuring the plasma potassium concentration at about three months will normally pick out those who do.

Hyperkalaemia is usually the consequence of giving potassium with a diuretic to a patient with poor renal function; giving a potassium supplement together with a distal tubular diuretic; or giving a distal tubular diuretic to a patient with renal failure. As a general rule neither distal tubular diuretics nor potassium supplements should be given to patients with renal failure. Combined diuretic and potassium tablets increase the risk that potassium will unthinkingly be prescribed for patients with poor renal function. Today's good renal function may be tomorrow's renal failure, and the appropriateness of a potassium supplement or the use of a distal tubular diuretic may change with time and intercurrent illness.

Hypercalcaemia and hypocalcaemia

Excessive dosage of vitamin D (or newer analogues) or of soluble calcium salts used as antacids (fortunately rarely used in Britain but common abroad) are the only likely causes of iatrogenic hypercalcaemia. The plasma calcium concentration must be watched at intervals of a month or two for as long[1] as pharmacological doses of vitamin D are given—and the indications for such treatment are few. A very large dose of vitamin D may be necessary in post-thyroidectomy hypoparathyroidism, for example, but the initially effective dose will almost invariably eventually cause hypercalcaemia (with nephrocalcinosis and renal failure) if not reduced at the right moment.

Osteomalacia sometimes develops in association with prolonged anticonvulsant treatment, especially in the elderly. Induction of increased hepatic hydroxylation of vitamin D is largely responsible, but the intestinal effects of vitamin D on calcium absorption may also be impaired. The symptoms are insidious and may be most disabling—weakness, bone pain, and pathological fractures—and they respond well to treatment with vitamin D; the symptoms must, however, be correctly diagnosed to be cured.

URATE METABOLISM

Diuretics increase plasma urate; thiazides by interfering with tubular secretion of urate, and all by reducing plasma volume. Plasma urate concentration should be measured before giving diuretics; it will be high in patients with chronic renal failure and in a few hypertensive patients. Gout is the obvious risk and is surprisingly rare in association with the hyperuricaemia of chronic renal failure, probably because rapid changes in concentration are more important than the absolute concentration itself; gouty interstitial nephritis is a less obvious danger, whose incidence is uncertain.

Acute attacks of gout may also be precipitated by allopurinol and other drugs that rapidly lower the plasma urate concentration. Cytotoxic drugs are apt to release sufficient nucleoprotein to produce a dramatic and dangerous rise in the plasma urate concentration (acute renal failure being the major hazard) and for that reason allopurinol is given as a prelude to chemotherapy.

CARBOHYDRATE METABOLISM

Drugs cause diabetes mellitus either, like thiazides, by interfering with release of insulin or, like adrenal corticosteroids, by opposing the actions of insulin. (Other mechanisms, such as the cytotoxic effects of the alkylating agent streptotozine on the pancreas, are outside the scope of this article.) Symptomatic hyperglycaemia may take years to develop, depending on initial glucose tolerance and perhaps age, or may appear within weeks as with diazoxide. So insidious may be the onset of symptoms and so chronic the treatment that has eventually caused them that diagnosis may be long delayed, and the cause of the maturity-onset diabetes may even escape detection altogether. Many oral contraceptives impair glucose tolerance but it has yet to be shown that the impairment is of practical consequence.

Although it is perhaps obvious that overdose of drugs designed to control metabolic disease—that is, antithyroid drugs or thyroxine—will produce the opposite disease, the danger of overactivity of long-acting hypoglycaemic agents, such as chlorpropamide, must be emphasised, especially in elderly patients and in those taking beta-adrenoceptor drugs, which impair the hepatic mobilisation of glucose in response to hypoglycaemia. Hypoglycaemic coma caused by chlorpropamide may be rare, but confusion and dementia are probably more prevalent than is realised. Long-acting insulins are likewise best avoided in the elderly.

Lactic acidosis, the result of lactate production exceeding its utilisation, is usually a byproduct of serious acute disease but it can be caused by intravenous fructose, sorbitol, and ethanol, and by drugs such as phenformin and metformin, especially in patients with renal, respiratory, or cardiac failure. These compounds should be avoided in such patients and used with caution in others.

CONCLUSION

Drug-induced metabolic disease is usually predictable and arises not out of ignorance but from failure to assess correctly the risks of a changing picture of disease, age, diet, or interactions with other treatment. Each move on the chessboard of treatment carries consequences that must be foreseen to be avoided.

Drug-induced haematological disease

AUDREY A DAWSON

The taunt about yesterday's remedies was that they were largely ineffectual. Today's treatment is often extremely effective but unfortunately has frequent bad effects, and much of modern therapeutic effort has to be directed at recognising and preventing morbidity from useful drugs.

One group of organs that suffers much from drug-induced ills is the blood and the blood-forming tissues. In many haematological textbooks there is a chapter on drug-induced blood diseases. It is unfortunately often true that in the ill effects produced by drugs on the blood, "the evil that men do lives after them; the good is oft interred with their bones." The effects may be predictable or unpredictable, and, indeed, drug-induced blood changes may be the first sign of unnoticed hereditary blood disorder, such as glucose-6-phosphate-dehydrogenase (G6PD) deficiency.

MARROW HYPOPLASIA

Drug-induced mild hypoplasia of the blood cells is used clinically as the guide to the maximum safe dosage of cytotoxic drugs in treating many forms of malignant disease; the blood cells are a convenient tissue to biopsy at frequent intervals. Such drugs will always cause marrow depression, although the dose required to do so will show enormous variation among people, and is modified considerably by such factors as previous radiotherapy and the presence of infection and malnutrition. Sometimes the nadir of the blood count is delayed, as with melphalan, and sometimes one element of the blood cells is depressed more than the others—for instance, the nitrosoureas affect particularly the platelet count. Long-continued bone marrow damage by cytotoxic agents can produce more subtle effects—for instance, in patients having adjuvant chemotherapy for breast carcinoma a late effect is persistent depression of the neutrophil polymorph precursors without a fall in the total white cell count. In fact, marrow aspirate in patients on cytotoxic chemotherapy with only modest depression of the peripheral blood count is often surprisingly hypocellular and fatty.

Some drugs, harmless to most people in the normal therapeutic dose, will occasionally at that dose cause aplastic anaemia. The best-known example is chloramphenicol, where the risk is to about 1 in 60 000 people exposed to it, and the same odds are probably true of phenylbutazone. There is no way of identifying before use people with such a susceptibility; the defect may be in the marrow cells, at different phases of cell development, or be a defect of detoxification or excretion of that drug.

Thrombocytopenia

Aplasia (or, much more commonly, hypoplasia) may affect all three elements of the blood—red cells, white cells, and platelets—or may affect one element mainly or alone. When only one element is affected an immune-complex process is probably concerned—for instance, in drug-induced thrombocytopenia, where antibody production can be shown in some cases and where abundant megakaryocytes can usually be found in the marrow. This was first noted with the hypnotic apronal (Sedormid); hence the old name "Sedormid purpura." Of the present-day drugs producing this immune thrombocytopenia, the anti-tuberculosis antibiotic rifampicin is an important occasional cause, and the thrombocytopenia of the thiazide diuretics, sulphonamides, digitoxin, quinidine, quinine, and parenteral penicillin probably has the same mechanism.

Neutropenia

Neutropenia may be caused by a direct toxic effect on the marrow as with cytotoxic drugs, or be an occasional finding in sensitive people. "Immune" neutropenia is less easy to prove than is thrombocytopenia, and many drugs have been incriminated. These include the anti-inflammatory drugs, especially phenylbutazone; antihistamines, such as chlorpheniramine; antithyroid drugs, such as methylthiouracil and carbimazole; antidiabetic drugs, such as tolbutamide and chlorpropamide; phenothiazines, such as chlorpromazine; various antibiotics, metronidazole, aminosalicylic acid, isoniazid, and the thiazides. The onset of neutropenia may be sudden, even in a patient who is well established taking the drug; and total agranulocytosis (absence of all mature cells of myeloid series from the blood) may occur, but is fairly rare, so that the old system of monitoring the white cell count of all patients taking, for example, antithyroid drugs, is probably not worth while. Chronic neutropenia, however, is not an uncommon cause of reference to a blood clinic, and drug-induced neutropenia must be among the commonest causes.

Acute myeloid leukaemia

Other effects of drugs on the white blood cells are less easy to measure. Depression of the normal functions of chemotaxis and phagocytosis by anti-inflammatory drugs has been shown. There is also considerable evidence that a marrow, once rendered hypoplastic after insult by a drug, is much more liable than normal to develop acute myeloid leukaemia. The major problem here is the impossibility of ascertaining how totally normal and stable the marrow was before the insult. There is a high index of suspicion about melphalan (an alkylating agent often used in myeloma) in inducing acute myeloid leukaemia, but in myeloma the marrow is already grossly abnormal, and several cases of simultaneous appearance of myeloma and acute leukaemia have been recorded. Similarly, the immunosuppressant drugs used during renal transplantation have been incriminated in the subsequent high risk of developing lymphomas; and the drugs used in Hodgkin's disease may have some part in the later risk of acute leukaemia, which is higher than expected in an age-matched population.

Dyserythropoiesis

Red cell hypoplasia alone is rare, but the red blood cell may show evidence of other forms of drug-induced marrow upset in the form of dyserythropoiesis. This may take several forms.

Megaloblastosis—Megaloblastosis with or without the development of megaloblastic anaemia is one form. Many drugs interfere with the absorption of vitamin B_{12} from the ileum, including neomycin, amino-salicylic acid, metformin, and various anticonvulsants. Although this results in a low serum vitamin B_{12} concentration, this rarely results in a definite megaloblastic anaemia. Nevertheless, a clinically important form of iatrogenic vitamin B_{12} deficiency recently described occurs in patients being artificially ventilated with a gaseous mixture containing 50% nitrous oxide, after cardiac bypass surgery, or in general intensive care. The picture, clinically and haematologically, is that of acute vitamin B_{12} deficiency, probably from interference by the nitrous oxide with B_{12} function due to oxidation.

Methotrexate and cytarabine are both powerful antifolates and cytotoxic agents. Many anticonvulsants, especially phenytoin, primidone, and barbiturates, produce folate deficiency, the incidence depending apparently on the dose and type of drug and the diet of the patient; relatively few patients develop severe megaloblastic anaemia. Trimethoprim, usually given as co-trimoxazole (Septrin), inhibits bacterial dihydrofolate reductase, and megaloblastic anaemia has been noted especially when co-trimoxazole has been used long term, and in patients with dietary folate deficiency. Pyrimethamine, related to trimethoprim chemically, may have the same effect. An important cause of acute megaloblastosis is hyperalimentation, usually using intravenous essential amino-acids, sorbitol, and ethanol. Postoperatively in a malnourished patient, often with gastrointestinal cancer, the condition is of considerable importance, because hypoplasia and disordered maturation affect all the marrow cells, and acute leucopenia and thrombocytopenia may result. This can be prevented by the simultaneous addition of daily intravenous folid acid.

Sideroblastic anaemia—Sideroblastic anaemia is another form of dyserythropoiesis that may be drug-induced. Here the biochemical lesion is not an abnormality of DNA synthesis in erythrocyte formation but a fundamental abnormality of haem development. In anti-tuberculosis treatment with isoniazid and cycloserine, after several months a small proportion of patients, perhaps with an underlying genetic tendency, develop a rapid fall in haemoglobin, with the marrow showing characteristic ring sideroblasts. Alcohol used therapeutically in hyperalimentation may also produce sideroblastosis.

Haemolytic anaemia

In megaloblastic and sideroblastic anaemias there is both reduced production and increased destruction of red cells, a mixture of hypoplasia and haemolysis. Certain drugs produce a pure haemolytic anaemia, however, and the number of drugs recognised as doing so is increasing.

Penicillin and many cephalosporins are small molecules, which produce IgG-type antibodies. The latter do not fix complement, and red blood cells that have been exposed to and coated with penicillin may lyse (modestly and extravascularly) when high doses of intravenous penicillin are given. These two groups of antibiotics are likely to cross-react in this as in other respects.

The more usual drug-induced haemolytic mechanism is: drug + serum protein + antibody → red blood cell reaction. When complement is added the red blood cells lyse, intravascularly, so that haemoglobinuria and sometimes renal failure occurs. Drugs in common use that occasionally produce this effect include quinine and quinidine, aminosalicylic acid, isoniazid, and the sulphonamides (including sulphasalazine).

One special form of drug-induced haemolytic anaemia is that associated with α-methyldopa treatment. Around 20% of patients treated with this drug for three months or more develop a positive direct antiglobulin test (Coombs test) of IgG-type showing rhesus-specificity. About 0·5% of all patients on the drug will develop overt haemolytic anaemia; the more antibody present in the serum the more likely is the patient to develop anaemia. Haemolysis may be severe enough to require blood transfusion and temporary use of corticosteroids. The drug should never be used again, even though haemolysis stops within a few weeks and the direct antiglobulin test reverts to negative in six to 18 months after cessation of the drug. Other drugs incriminated in producing the same effect are chlordiazepoxide, mefenamic acid, flufenamic acid, and indomethacin; levodopa may produce the positive Coombs test.

Drug-induced haemolysis may occur when the red cell is already abnormal—for instance, in G6PD deficiency, which accounts for about 95% of all hereditary red cell metabolic defects. The incidence of this deficiency is widespread, being found in natives of China and Western Europe, as well as around the Mediterranean littoral and in negroes, so that, in multiracial Britain, it is a condition to be borne in mind. There are many different isoenzymes of G6PD (which is carried on the X chromosome, and has, thus, sex-linked inheritance), and different clinical features result from different isoenzyme deficiencies. The characteristic, however, of a G6PD-deficient red cell is that it haemolyses on exposure to oxidising stress, and the oxidant is often a drug.

Many drugs have been implicated in precipitating a haemolytic crisis in G6PD deficiency. Primaquin and the other antimalarials were the first drugs noted, but sulphonamides (including sulphasalazine and sulphamethoxazole or co-trimoxazole), various antibiotics such as nitrofurantoin, aminosalicylic acid, and isoniazid, and vitamin K analogues such as Synkavit have the same effect. Infection, bacterial or viral, may also cause acute haemolysis in susceptible people, and it has proved difficult to sort out the role of infection from that of drugs, such as aspirin-containing analgesics taken for symptomatic relief, in causing haemolysis. In any one patient with a particular isoenzyme deficiency many drugs may cause no haemolysis at all. The characteristic of this form of drug-induced haemolysis is that it stops after a few days, despite continuing the drug, as young red cells are entering the circulation.

Heinz bodies can often be shown in acute haemolysis. They result from precipitation of the globin chain of haemoglobin, because of oxidant stress in vivo. Heinz bodies reduce the ability of the red cell membrane to deform, so these red cells are delayed in the reticulo-endothelial system, allowing them to be haemolysed and phagocytosed, usually in the spleen. Their presence makes an easy laboratory method of showing oxidant damage to haemoglobin by drugs.

Chronic posthaemorrhagic anaemia

Probably the most common drug-induced haematological condition is chronic posthaemorrhagic anaemia resulting from taking aspirin or aspirin-containing drugs, often self-prescribed, and causing occult peptic bleeding. Aspirin can produce such an anaemia in two ways—by local irritation of the gastric mucosa and by fundamental and life-long damage to circulating platelets. Thus the effect of two aspirin tablets may be shown by in-vitro platelet function tests for at least a week. Most of the anti-inflammatory agents used in chronic painful joint conditions may also produce gastric erosions or occult peptic blood loss. Many patients have indigestion or occult bleeding or both (and these two problems are often disassociated) with one anti-inflammatory drug, but none with another. Gastroduodenal blood loss may be much more overt and acute with any of these drugs.

Haemostatic defects

The production of haemostatic defects by drugs tends to be intentional and the main action, as with the oral anticoagulants (warfarin, coumarin, and the indanedione derivatives), the parenteral anticoagulants—for instance, heparin—and the drugs producing controlled defibrination, such as streptokinase and ancrod. Drugs such as aspirin and dipyrimadole are now being considered in the prophylaxis of further arterial thrombosis both after myocardial infarction and in transient ischaemic cerebral episodes. Thrombocytopenia has been mentioned earlier.

Lastly, some drugs will affect the blood in its role of monitor to the health of the body. Eosinophilia, and sometimes basophilia, may occur as indications of allergy, where perhaps the target organ of the drug is the skin. Similarly, the LE cell phenomenon can be shown in the blood of some patients having procainamide and hydrallazine, and these patients often develop the systemic features of systemic lupus erythematosus.

Drug-induced disease has been particularly well demonstrated with regard to the blood cells because of the ease in biopsying these cells. This has led to daunting lists of drugs that may upset blood cells, and since blood is such a complicated organ, the difficulty is often to unravel the mechanism of the damage.

Drug-induced gastrointestinal disease

P L ZENTLER-MUNRO, T C NORTHFIELD

Surveys of hospital inpatients show that 20–40% of all side effects of drugs affect the gastrointestinal tract. Because most drugs are taken by mouth, patients tend to blame medication for their gastrointestinal symptoms; nearly all oral drugs have gastrointestinal side effects. Gastrointestinal symptoms are important because they may reduce patient compliance, and also because they may herald the development of a drug-induced disease. In this article attention will be restricted to specific gastrointestinal diseases attributed to drugs. Usually, these diseases have pathological changes that do not resolve immediately the drug is withdrawn.

MOUTH

Aspirin, potassium supplements, corticosteroids, pancreatic enzyme tablets, and sublingual isoprenaline cause ulceration of the buccal mucosa if the tablets are sucked. Patients, especially children, should be advised to swallow tablets with water. Buccal ulceration may also occur as part of a generalised hypersensitivity reaction, the most severe form being the Stevens-Johnson syndrome. When drug-induced, usually after sulphonamides, barbiturates, or penicillin, it responds to withdrawal of the drug.

Bone marrow suppression induced by antimitotic drugs, carbimazole, or chloramphenicol may present first as buccal ulceration or as petechial haemorrhage or infection within the mouth. Herpetic ulcers are common during immunosuppressive treatment. Oral candidiasis may complicate treatment with antibiotics, corticosteroids (including inhaled beclamethasone), or immunosuppressive agents.

OESOPHAGUS

Candidiasis may also effect the oesophagus and can cause dysphagia. It may not be suspected clinically if the mouth is not affected, but can be diagnosed endoscopically or radiologically. There are many reports of oesophageal ulceration and structure formation from slow-release potassium chloride tablets; in some cases a tablet has been found adjacent to the ulcer, providing strong evidence for a causal relationship. Other drugs may cause ulceration in the absence of any oesophageal abnormality, including aspirin and the newer non-steroidal anti-inflammatory analgesics, emepronium bromide, doxycycline, and slow-release preparations of iron and quinidine. Patients should swallow such preparations with water, and should not lie down immediately afterwards.

Drugs known to cause mucosal damage should not be given in conditions where there may be a delay in oesophageal emptying, as in oesophageal stricture, scleroderma, enlargement of the left atrium, or immediately after cardiac surgery.

Symptomatic gastro-oesophageal reflux may occur with anti-Parkinsonian drugs of the anticholinergic group, which are known to decrease lower oesophageal sphincter pressure.

STOMACH

Peptic ulcer has been reported in association with many drugs, but as it is common in the general population it can be expected to occur at least as commonly in patients taking drugs. The incidence of peptic ulcer is said to be higher in patients with rheumatoid arthritis, irrespective of treatment, than in the general population; this has given the drugs used to treat rheumatoid arthritis—salicylates, corticosteroids, and the non-steroidal anti-inflammatory analgesics—a notoriety they may not deserve.

Surveys in Australia and the USA have shown that women with chronic gastric ulcers consume more salicylate than control subjects attending outpatient clinics with non-ulcer dyspepsia; no difference has been found for men or for patients with duodenal ulcers. Other surveys have shown that patients with major gastrointestinal haemorrhage consume more salicylate than patients admitted to hospital for any other reason. This association is strongest with chronic continuous salicylate use. Salicylate-induced haemorrhage occurs more often from acute erosions than from chronic peptic ulcer. Salicylates increase the rate of occult blood loss in patients with peptic ulcer and in healthy controls. The incidence of such occult blood loss does not correlate with the incidence of major ulcer haemorrhage. Dispersed ("soluble") and buffered aspirin cause less occult blood loss than acetylsalicylic acid, and gastric erosion appears to be rarer with enteric-coated aspirin. Although the exact relation between salicylate and gastric disease is still disputed, it seems sensible not to prescribe salicylates to patients with gastric ulcer or dyspepsia, or to those who have previously suffered dyspepsia or gastrointestinal bleeding with salicylates.

Corticosteroids have long been reputed to cause peptic ulcer. An analysis of 42 double-blind controlled trials of steroids in the treatment of a variety of diseases including rheumatoid arthritis has shown no difference in the incidence of dyspepsia or gastrointestinal haemorrhage between active and placebo groups. In studies where a history of peptic ulcer was common, and did not exclude patients from the trial, there was no evidence of reactivation in the group taking steroids. These epidemiological data are consistent with experimental evidence that steroids do not increase occult gastrointestinal blood loss or cause gastric erosions.

Phenylbutazone and indomethacin commonly cause dyspepsia in patients with rheumatoid arthritis. Despite many case reports of peptic ulceration and perforation in patients treated with these drugs, controlled studies have not confirmed the common belief that these complications are more common in patients treated with phenylbutazone or indomethacin than in patients treated with other drugs.

The many newer non-steroidal anti-inflammatory analgesics appear to be better tolerated than salicylates in patients with a previous history of dyspepsia. Each drug claims to have a lower incidence of unwanted effects than its competitors; but unfortunately the trials on which claims are based seldom choose appropriate dosages for such comparisons. Gastrointestinal haemorrhage has been reported during treatment with each of these drugs and is said to be particularly common with naproxen. No systemic investigation of the incidence of peptic ulcer and gastrointestinal haemorrhage has been performed, but one study in progress suggests that these drugs may be more commonly associated with haematemesis and melaena than salicylate. The non-steroidal anti-inflammatory analgesics are all more expensive than aspirin, and many are less potent. They should therefore be reserved for patients who develop dyspepsia while taking soluble aspirin. Patients who have been shown to have a peptic ulcer should if possible be treated with an analgesic such as paracetamol, which has no anti-inflammatory action.

SMALL INTESTINE

Ulceration, perforation, and stricture of the small intestine are now well-recognised complications of enteric-coated potassium chloride tablets. All preparations containing enteric-coated potassium chloride have now been withdrawn, but the introduction of a slow-release preparation has not abolished the problem. Since 1970 there have been several reports of mid-ileal ulcers and strictures in patients taking Slow K. Compound tablets containing a diuretic and slow-release potassium chloride have also been implicated. It seems sensible therefore to use potassium-sparing diuretics when the small intestine is abnormal.

Paralytic ileus may be induced by anticholinergic drugs (including anti-Parkinsonian drugs of this class), tricyclic antidepressants, phenothiazines, and opiates. Tricyclic antidepressants and clonidine can also cause the syndrome of intestinal pseudo-obstruction; recognition of this can save patients from an unnecessary laparotomy. Both conditions resolve on withdrawal of the offending drug.

Infarction of the small intestine due to thrombosis of the superior mesenteric artery has been reported many times in women taking high-dose oestrogen-containing oral contraceptives. This severe and irreversible catastrophe is otherwise extremely rare in young women; its attribution to the oral contraceptive is consistent with oestrogen-induced thrombosis elsewhere. Thrombosis of the coeliac artery, inferior mesenteric artery, hepatic vein, and portal vein have also been reported.

Drugs can cause malabsorption in several ways, and this may lead to failure of concurrent medication. Several drugs inhibit pancreatic lipase, but only mefenamic acid has been reported to cause steatorrhoea. Neomycin and cholestyramine bind bile acids leading to malabsorption of fat and fat-soluble vitamins. Neomycin can also damage the enterocyte and reduce disaccharidase activity; at high doses partial villous atrophy may ensue. Colchicine and antimitotic drugs reduce cell turnover in all rapidly dividing tissues. They can cause partial villous atrophy during treatment, with restoration of normal architecture between courses.

Many drugs interfere with absorption or transport of vitamin B_{12} but only neomycin, cholestyramine, para-aminosalicylic acid, isoniazid, and metformin have been reported to cause anaemia by this mechanism. Anaemia from malabsorption of folic acid is common in long-continued anticonvulsant treatment, particularly with phenytoin. Folic acid malabsorption has been reported with the oral contraceptive but does not cause anaemia unless the diet is inadequate.

LARGE INTESTINE

Broad-spectrum antibiotics cause diarrhoea in up to 30% of patients. With some antibiotics, such as ampicillin, the diarrhoea is attributed to an alteration in colonic flora. Diarrhoea after treatment with antibiotics usually improves when the drug is withdrawn, as does that due to other drugs such as magnesium containing antacids, iron salts, guanethidine, and methyldopa.

Diarrhoea that persists after withdrawal of antibiotics may signal the development of pseudomembranous colitis. This disease was rare before the introduction of antibiotics. It first became widely recognised as a common and potentially lethal complication of treatment with lincomycin and clindamycin in the early 1970s. Ampicillin, penicillin, sulphonamides, chloramphenicol, and tetracycline also cause this syndrome, although less often than lincomycin and clindamycin. The diagnosis should be considered in a patient who develops persistent diarrhoea after any antibiotic. The disease appears to be particularly common when antibiotics are used after colonic surgery; signs of septicaemia and pelvic sepsis may falsely suggest a breakdown of the anastomosis. Recognition of the disease can save the patient from unnecessary surgery or even death. Pseudomembranous colitis may start during treatment with an antibiotic, or up to two weeks after stopping it. It may present as mild diarrhoea, or as an acute fulminant colitis. Sigmoidoscopy is usually diagnostic and should never be omitted, however ill the patient. The characteristic appearance is of raised plaques with a specific histological appearance. Barium enema may show characteristic changes but is dangerous in fulminant cases. Pseudomembranous colitis is now thought to be caused by overgrowth of *Clostridium difficile* in the colon, with production of a necrotising toxin. Both the organism and the toxin can be detected in the stool and may distinguish pseudomembranous colitis from non-specific post-antibiotic diarrhoea. A recent controlled trial has shown that vancomycin, a non-absorbed antibiotic to which this organism is sensitive, rapidly improves the condition of the patient, reverses the sigmoidoscopic appearances, and eliminates the organism and its toxin from the stool.

Staphylococcal enterocolitis is an extremely rare but severe complication of broad-spectrum antibiotic treatment and may be complicated by septicaemia, portal pyaemia, and metastatic abscesses.

The oral contraceptive can cause a severe form of ischaemic colitis that is otherwise extremely rare in young women. Unlike the infarction due to arterial thrombosis affecting the small intestine, this complication may resolve on withdrawal of the drug.

Laxative abuse is sometimes not suspected as a cause of chronic diarrhoea, because patients do not realise that their consumption of purgatives is excessive, or because they deliberately conceal it. Diarrhoea may be accompanied by weakness due to hypokalaemia, which if prolonged may lead to renal impairment. The anthraquinone laxatives (senna, cascara), phenolphthalein, and magnesium sulphate are commonly responsible and may be detected by appropriate tests. Barium enema appearances of a dilated featureless colon may suggest ulcerative colitis, but characteristically the changes are most pronounced in the ascending colon and transient pseudostrictures may be seen on screening. Rectal histology may be normal or may show pigmentation (melanosis coli) with anthraquinone cathartics. In long-standing cases permanent damage to the myenteric plexus may cause persistent diarrhoea, which is best treated by faecal bulking agents.

PANCREAS

Many drugs have been reported to cause acute pancreatitis on the basis that recurrent attacks cease when the offending drug is withdrawn. The evidence is strongest for corticosteroids. Focal pancreatitis is more common in necropsies of steroid-treated patients than matched controls. The incidence of acute pancreatitis in children with the nephrotic syndrome is reported to be greater in those treated with steroids. In patients treated with steroids the symptoms and signs of pancreatitis are often suppressed, and the prognosis is poor even if the drug can be withdrawn. Pancreatitis is often identified as the cause of death only at necropsy. Its incidence in steroid-treated patients is unrelated to the dose or duration of treatment.

Acute pancreatitis has been reported in women taking oral contraceptives, and responds to withdrawal of the drug. Thiazides, sulphonamides, clofibrate, methyldopa, and guanethidine are the other main drugs reported to cause acute pancreatitis. A careful drug history should always be taken in pancreatitis, and withdrawal of all drugs should be attempted.

MISCELLANEOUS

Clofibrate and oestrogen-containing oral contraceptives increase the cholesterol saturation of bile. The incidence of gall stones is increased in patients treated with these drugs.

Sclerosing peritonitis is now a well-recognised complication of treatment with practolol. It has not been reported with any other beta-blocker apart from one dubious report with oxprenolol. Methysergide causes retroperitoneal fibrosis that may lead to narrowing of the colon or mesenteric vessels, but it is rarely used nowadays.

CONCLUSION

The list presented in this article comprises only the commoner and better documented drug-induced gastrointestinal diseases. Gastrointestinal symptoms are common with oral medication, and a detailed drug history should always be taken. The possibility of a drug reaction should not be dismissed simply because such an effect has not been reported; neither should it be accepted simply because the patient reports symptoms immediately after starting treatment. Whenever possible a drug under suspicion should be withdrawn, but some drug-induced diseases may need specific treatment (particularly pseudomembranous colitis). Most drugs should be taken with meals and all should be swallowed with water.

Drug-induced liver disease

P W N KEELING, R P H THOMPSON

In about 8% of reports of adverse drug reactions the liver is affected, although deaths are unusual. The liver is central in the metabolism and excretion of many drugs. Metabolism inactivates them, but some, such as cyclophosphamide and paracetamol, are converted in the liver into toxic intermediate metabolites. In general, drug metabolism proceeds in two phases, both catalysed by enzymes in the membranes of the endoplasmic reticulum in the cell.[1] The first is of oxidation, reduction, or hydrolysis, the second of conjugation with glucuronic acid, amino-acids, or sulphate. Larger, more water-soluble (polar) compounds are the end result, the larger being excreted into bile, the smaller into urine. Although there are differences between the activities of metabolising enzymes in cells in different parts of the hepatic lobule, it is not generally possible to relate these to the site of damage in the hepatic lobule produced by drugs.

PREDICTABLE (DIRECT) HEPATOTOXINS

Liver cell necrosis

A few drugs and chemicals, such as ferrous sulphate excess, tannic acid, paracetamol excess, tetrachloroethylene, aspirin, cytotoxic drugs, and tetracycline excess, predictably produce necrosis of liver cells—namely a hepatitis—when given in sufficient dosage to man and many animals. Young animals are often more resistant.

Tannic acid caused liver damage when applied to burns from the surface of which it was absorbed, and mild liver damage has been reported after barium enemas to which tannic acid had been added to improve coating of the mucosa. The drug is itself hepatotoxic, without undergoing metabolic transformation to an active molecule.

Tetracyclines—Large doses of tetracyclines have produced in animals and man a strange, often fatal liver disease, in which there is infiltration of the liver with fat but little necrosis of liver cells. The liver damage occurs chiefly in pregnant women, particularly those with renal failure. Tetracyclines have widespread poisonous effects on cellular metabolism, and this presumably underlies this toxicity.

Fusidic acid, particularly given intravenously, can sometimes cause jaundice.

Paracetamol is transformed into a toxic metabolite.[2] It is rapidly removed from the blood into liver cells, where chiefly glucuronic acid and sulphate conjugates are formed that pass into urine. Minor amounts are oxidised to metabolites that combine with the sulphur-containing glutathione. Although therapeutic doses are therefore harmless, overdoses (25 g or more) cause severe liver damage, since the huge load of drug saturates these normal detoxification pathways. There is then intracellular accumulation of toxic metabolites, and they bind to membranes and irreversibly damage them and their enzymes. This knowledge has led to a rational treatment of paracetamol poisoning with sulphur compounds, such as cysteamine, acetylcysteine, and methionine. The degree of liver cell damage depends on the dose of paracetamol and also the rate of its absorption, since this determines the rate at which it is presented to the liver.

Tetrachloroethylene can damage the liver by a similar mechanism.

Recently mild hepatotoxicity has been reported in patients with rheumatological diseases taking large doses of aspirin, and the high frequency of this reaction suggests that it is a direct toxic effect.

Cytotoxic drugs, such as azathioprine and mercaptopurine, have caused liver damage in a few patients, even though these drugs are sometimes given to treat chronic liver disease. Cholestasis also occasionally occurs in patients with renal disease treated with azathioprine.

Cholestasis

Careful studies have shown that oestrogens administered to women in amounts no larger than those secreted during pregnancy regularly produce impairment of the secretion of bile and of excretion of the dye sulphobromophthalein sodium into bile; that is, they cause cholestasis.[3] In a few women the contraceptive pill invariably produces itching, and less often reversible jaundice, and in a minority of these women a similar cholestasis always develops during the last trimester of pregnancy. This hepatic reaction is thought to be an exaggerated response to the oestrogen component.

Some other groups of patients are also abnormally sensitive to oestrogens—namely, those with primary biliary cirrhosis (chronic, destructive, non-suppurative cholangitis) or with the rare congenital Dublin-Johnson and benign recurrent cholestatic syndromes. They develop jaundice.

Large doses of anabolic steroids and some androgens also invariably produce a mild cholestasis and, in a few patients, jaundice. Patients with primary biliary cirrhosis are again more susceptible, and most of them when given norethandrolone to relieve itching become more jaundiced.

So far the molecular structure of all these cholestatic drugs has included a 17α-alkyl-substituted group. The mechanism of the effect is unknown, although oestrogens may increase the permeability of the wall of the bile canaliculi so that water leaks out of bile, concentrating it, and leading to stagnation in these tiny intercellular channels.

Drug-induced liver disease

UNPREDICTABLE HEPATIC REACTIONS

A large and increasing number of drugs have caused liver damage varying from mild hepatitis, cholestasis, or granuloma formation to fatal hepatic necrosis.[4,5] Generalised signs of hypersensitivity, such as rashes, arthralgia, and eosinophilia, are also sometimes seen. The reactions are unpredictable, and occur in only a few patients taking the drug, usually within the first weeks of treatment. These unusually susceptible patients may have some underlying immunological defect, or they may have an inherited abnormality of the hepatic enzymes metabolising the drug. The hepatic damage is often classified into hepatitis or cholestasis, but these may be difficult to separate.

Hepatitis (see table)

Widespread necrosis of liver cells and release from them of aminotransferase (transaminase) enzymes into blood has been seen with several psychiatric drugs, among which iproniazid caused the highest frequency of deaths relative to the amount of drug prescribed.

Drugs causing unpredictable hepatitis

Monoamine oxidase inhibitors	Penicillin
Antituberculosis drugs	Chlordiazepoxide
Anaesthetic agents	Phenindione
Phenytoin	

Antituberculosis drugs[4,6]—The mechanism of the hepatic reactions antituberculosis drugs may cause is complex. Firstly, serious liver damage after taking isoniazid, para-aminosalicylic acid, rifampicin, ethambutol, and pyrazinamide is rare. Many more patients develop mildly raised levels of aminotransferases during the first few weeks of treatment with isoniazid and rifampicin, but spontaneously improve if treatment is continued.

Hepatotoxicity may be due to an abnormal accumulation and binding to cellular membranes of one of its metabolites in the liver—that is, a direct toxic effect. Abnormal results of liver function tests seem to be more common when both rifampicin and isoniazid are given together to older patients, and possibly to those with pre-existing chronic liver disease or to alcoholics.

Thirdly, rifampicin reversibly impairs bilirubin metabolism and in some patients raises blood levels of unconjugated bilirubin; this may falsely suggest to the doctor that serious liver damage is developing.

Finally, rifampicin induces drug-metabolising enzymes in the liver, and probably therefore increases the rate of its own metabolism and that of isoniazid. This may explain why results of liver function tests are usually most abnormal in the first weeks of treatment, and later improve, and why rifampicin may increase the frequency of isoniazid hepatitis.

Postanaesthetic hepatitis—Abnormal results of liver function tests, and occasionally jaundice and fatal liver failure mimicking viral hepatitis, can follow anaesthesia and surgery, but controversy surrounds the role in this of anaesthesia in general versus halothane in particular. Transient impairment of liver function is more common after halothane than other anaesthetics, but it is important to balance this against the knowledge that halothane is a safe anaesthetic and the most used. Abnormal results of liver function tests and raised levels of serum enzymes have long been known to follow any anaesthetic, however brief, but there is more concern about the infrequent occurrence of severe liver failure that may develop about a week after anaesthesia. There is now plausible evidence that this hepatic reaction is more common in the obese, and when halothane anaesthetics are given repeatedly at intervals of less than a month.

The reaction was thought to be a hypersensitive one, but there is increasing evidence that halothane can be metabolised, especially by the hypoxic liver, to hepatotoxic metabolites. Immunological sensitivity to halothane has also been found in patients tested after an episode of postanaesthetic jaundice.

Granulomatous hepatitis

Localised areas of liver cell damage and collections of histiocytes (granulomas) have been found within the hepatic lobules of a few patients taking various drugs, such as phenylbutazone, halothane, sulphonamides, and allopurinol, of which phenylbutazone is the best recorded. This reaction is seldom severe, although deaths have been reported.

Unpredictable cholestasis

Some drugs, such as phenothiazines, iprindole, chlorpropamide, thiouracil, erythromycin estolate, and gold, produce a selective cholestasis in a few patients taking them.

Phenothiazines, especially chlorpromazine, have a particularly bad reputation, and some abnormalities of liver function occur in a large minority of patients taking them, although jaundice is rare. The mechanism is not known, but in animal experiments chlorpromazine has various effects on the liver, including an impairment of excretion of sulphobromophthalein sodium, so it may prove to be a direct hepatotoxin.

In occasional patients jaundice is prolonged for months, and the development of cirrhosis and death have been reported. The jaundice usually develops within a few weeks of starting the drug, but we are sceptical of suggestions that a single tablet can induce it.

Erythromycin—Although the estolate ester has long been reported to cause cholestasis, recent reports have emphasised that other forms of the antibiotic can also do so.

Chronic hepatitis and cirrhosis [2 4]

Until recently it was believed that chronic hepatitis, in which chronic inflammatory cells infiltrate the portal tracts of the liver and raised levels of hepatic enzymes are found in blood, did not occur from drug-induced liver damage, even though prolonged intake of alcohol, for instance, readily causes the disease. It is now clear, however, that a few drugs such as oxyphenisatin, methyldopa, nitrofurantoin, methotrexate, and vitamin A excess may be implicated. The liver recovers when they are withdrawn.

Oxyphenisatin—This laxative was fortunately not much used in Britain, but it has been associated with chronic hepatitis in other European countries and in North America and Australia. Such an association is easily overlooked, and was for a long time, so that there may be other drugs and environmental toxins that can cause non-virus-associated chronic liver damage.

Methyldopa and *nitrofurantoin* are also implicated.

Methotrexate—Chronic fibrosis of the liver follows prolonged administration of methotrexate, usually given for severe psoriasis, but the frequency of this is uncertain since many patients have also admitted heavy alcohol intake. The concomitant portal hypertension is not always reversible on withdrawing the drug.

OTHER HEPATIC REACTIONS

Hepatic vein thrombosis

Obstruction of the large hepatic veins draining the liver causes rapid enlargement of the liver, ascites, and often liver failure—the Budd-Chiari syndrome. The incidence of this rare syndrome is greater than expected in women taking the contraceptive pill,[3] as are thromboses elsewhere in the body.

Peliosis hepatis

Lately there have been reports of this unusual lesion, which consists of dilated sinusoidal vessels and multiple blood cysts in the liver, developing in patients who have been receiving either anabolic steroids or the contraceptive pill.[3] It regresses on stopping treatment, but may present as an acute abdominal emergency from rupture of the liver.

Hepatic tumours[7]

Benign liver cell tumours have been reported in a few patients taking oral contraceptives or androgens, and these may also rupture. There is also suspicion that malignant hepatomas occur more often in these patients. Hepatomas and haemangioendotheliomas developed in patients 15–20 years after receiving the *x*-ray contrast medium thorium dioxide (Thorotrast), but new cases are now rare.

Porphyria

Many drugs precipitate crises in patients with the rare disease acute intermittent porphyria. Barbiturates seem particularly dangerous, but also anticonvulsants, sedatives, and griseofulvin. The mechanism appears to be induction in liver cells of the rate-limiting enzyme of the porphyrin pathway, aminolaevulinic acid (ALA) synthetase. Great excesses of the toxic porphyrin precursors ALA and porphobilinogen are then synthesised, and accumulate in the body because of a defect in the further conversion of porphobilinogen to uroporphyrin.

Gall stones

A clear association between the prevalence of gall stones and the administration of clofibrate has emerged[8] in recent trials of this agent in the prevention of coronary artery thrombosis. This may be because, as well as lowering blood cholesterol, clofibrate increases cholesterol and decreases bile acid excretion into bile.

In recent animal experiments oestrogens decreased the synthesis of bile acids in the liver; this would tend to reduce the solubility of cholesterol in bile, and may help to explain the association of gall stones with the female sex and the contraceptive pill.

MANAGEMENT OF HEPATIC DRUG REACTIONS

There are now few drugs that have not at some time been incriminated in the development of abnormal results of liver function tests, particularly in the correspondence columns of medical journals. So what does the doctor do when faced with a patient with increasingly abnormal test results and whom he finds has taken one or more potentially hepatotoxic drugs?

The patterns of liver function tests are too variable to help unless the aminotransferases are greatly raised. The histological appearance of liver biopsy specimens have lately been clearly reviewed.[9] Features favouring a drug lesion included a severe histological lesion relative to the clinical state of the patient, granulomas, and infiltration with eosinophils. These appearances, however, are not diagnostic, though they should exclude some other causes of jaundice, such as gall stones.

The doctor also has to balance the possible benefits of treatment against the real, if small, risk of fatal liver failure. If an equal, alternative treatment is available, such as for a hypotensive drug, this should be given. Indeed, there is seldom any place for a trial re-exposure of the drug. With antituberculosis treatment it seems wise to investigate liver function in patients not rapidly improving with treatment, or who develop nausea or increasing fever. Treatment can be continued if transaminase levels remain below an arbitrary level of three times raised and if one's nerves hold out, but if more than this treatment may have to be changed, even though the options for effective drugs are then so much reduced.

The diagnosis of postanaesthetic jaundice is difficult, although if severe it includes considerably raised aminotransferase levels, abnormal clotting, and liver failure with encephalopathy. If a patient has developed abnormal liver function or jaundice after a previous anaesthetic a non-halothane anaesthetic should preferably be given if the interval between anaesthetics is less than a month. If halothane is required a senior anaesthetist should administer it knowing the small risk that is entailed.

Attempts have been made to differentiate the total clinical picture of drug-induced hepatitis from viral hepatitis by entering the clinical and biochemical data into a computer model. Diagnosis is improved, but the model is not yet reliable enough to relieve the doctor of often difficult decisions.

This article has strictly adhered to the title and has therefore not discussed the effects of toxins, such as alcohol, on the liver, nor physiological defects of bilirubin metabolism produced by drugs, nor the general effects of induction of hepatic enzymes by drugs.

PWNK is an MRC Training Fellow.

REFERENCES

1 Williams RT. Hepatic metabolism of drugs. *Gut* 1972;**13**:579–85.
2 Mitchell JR, Nelson S, Thorgeirsson SS, *et al.* In Popper H, Schaffner F. *Progress in liver disease*. New York; Grune and Stratton, 1978;259–79
3 Anonymous. Oral contraceptives and the liver. *Br Med J* 1974; iv:430–1.
4 Black M. Hepatotoxicity: pathogenesis and therapeutic intervention. *Clin Gastroenterol* 1979;**8**:89–104.
5 Ludwig J. Drug effects on the liver. *Digestive Diseases and Sciences* 1979;**24**: 785–96.
6 Anonymous. Antituberculous drugs and the liver. *Br Med J* 1975; ii:522–3.
7 Anonymous. Liver tumours and the steroid hormoes. *Lancet* 1973;ii:1481.
8 Anonymous. Clofibrate: a final verdict. *Lancet* 1978;ii:1131–2.
9 Anonymous. Guidelines for diagnosis of therapeutic drug-induced liver injury in liver biopsies. *Lancet* 1974;i:854–7.

Preoperative assessment of patients

J NORMAN

Anaesthesia is a necessary evil. Necessary because without it surgery would be virtually impossible as would be a considerable number of investigations. Evil because it entails using drugs that make the patient defenceless. Alternative methods such as acupuncture, hypnosis, and electrical anaesthesia are not sufficiently reliable to replace inhaled or injected drugs.

When rendering a patient defenceless the anaesthetist takes on the responsibility of keeping the patient alive and bringing him back to normal function once the operation is over. The safety of modern anaesthesia reflects the skills used. In surveying ten years' operating at Groote Schuur hospital, Harrison[1] reported that with some 240 483 operations anaesthesia had caused death in only 53 patients, an incidence of 1 : 4537. Anaesthesia for caesarean section is always thought to present additional risks. The latest report on confidential inquiries into maternal deaths[2] indicated that the death rate from anaesthesia was 1 : 5933. The causes of death, and presumably of morbidity as well, have been well recognised: problems with breathing, problems with blood volume and cardiac function, and, more rarely, problems of adverse responses to drugs.

The essence of good anaesthetic care is to recognise when problems are likely to occur. Indeed, training may be regarded as taking three stages: in the first the trainee gets into trouble; in the second he learns to get out of trouble; and, finally, he learns to avoid trouble. One of the functions of the anaesthetist when seeing patients before operation is to assess the possibilities of problems and to plan accordingly. The cynic[3] may reduce the assessment to three questions: who is the surgeon, where is the patient going afterwards, and what is the operation. Even so, Fisher[3] states that the preoperative examination tells you "how and when." These are vital.

The basis for assessing a patient for anaesthetic and surgery must be to consider the responses likely to be seen with the particular operation for that patient in his state of health. The results will determine the choice of anaesthetic techniques and, perhaps, the planned postoperative management—whether as a day case or in an intensive care unit.

ASSESSMENT OF FITNESS FOR RISKS OF ANAESTHESIA AND SURGERY

It seems logical to expect that the more the patient is incapable of coping with the demands of normal physical activity the more likely he will be at risk from anaesthesia and surgery. One widely used assessment is that of the American Society of Anesthesiologists[4]—(I) normal healthy patient; (II) mild systemic disease; (III) severe systemic disease limiting activity but not incapacitating; (IV) incapacitating systemic disease with a constant threat to life; and (V) moribund, not expected to live 24 hours with or without surgery.

In a large series Dripps *et al*[5] found that the classification did give a general prediction as to the outcome. Nevertheless, the classification does not always detect the specific risks to the patient. The risks of developing a cardiac complication threatening life have been assessed by Goldman *et al.*[6] The main hazards that could be assessed before operation were a history of a myocardial infarction within the past six months and the presence of heart failure and any arrhythmia. Remarkably, the presence of angina by itself or hypertension did not predict the development of problems, although their series did not contain patients with severe hypertension. Milledge and Nunn[7] looked at patients with chronic obstructive airway disease and found that most did not develop problems apart from those who were in respiratory failure with a high carbon dioxide tension. For liver disease, Pugh *et al*[8] have developed a scoring system to predict the outcome over the subsequent year, using the presence of encephalopathy, bilirubinaemia, prolongation of the prothrombin time, and a low blood albumin concentration. These types of assessment will become more common for they consider the results of the total effects of surgery and anaesthesia.

Most anaesthetists ask for the haemoglobin concentration to be measured before surgery and will not readily anaesthetise patients if it is less than 10 g/dl. This is not because anaemic patients are more at risk but rather that, in Britain, there must be a cause for this degree of anaemia. Preoperative diagnosis and treatment can restore a normal haemoglobin concentration. Alternatively, if major surgery is imperative blood transfusions before and during surgery can be given.

SPECIFIC ANAESTHETIC PROBLEMS

One can almost construct an alphabet of potential problems for the anaesthetist which can be detected preoperatively.

Airways pose many problems. Difficulties in maintaining a clear airway may be expected in patients with various congenital defects: large goitres, full stomachs, or intestinal obstruction in pregnant patients, and many others.

Anaesthetics—Previous anaesthetics may also have produced their own problems—from postoperative nausea and vomiting through awareness to such major hazards as the development of malignant hyperthermia or hepatic failure. A history of what happened before is necessary as is an inquiry whether other members of the family have had problems.

Breathing or, more strictly, ventilation may cause problems in those with chronic respiratory failure or with muscular or neuromuscular disease, and in some with neurological disorders.

Circulation—This needs both taking a history to assess the risks of myocardial infarction and of rheumatic fever and an examination to detect heart failure and arrhythmias. The common cause of operative problems is shock. The presence of a blood volume or inadequate cardiac function must be detected.

Drugs that patients take can cause problems, although with most, if the anaesthetist knows what is being taken, there will be no problems. With most antihypertensive regimens the risks of stopping them because of possible dangers during anaesthesia and surgery are less than those of untreated hypertension and of stopping the drugs. Most anaesthetists will now want such treatment continued up to, during, and after the operation.

Endocrine disorders, such as diabetes, may cause trouble. Diabetes in particular needs careful management, especially in the unstable undergoing major surgery. Alberti and Thomas[9] have reviewed these problems.

Electrolyte disturbances are common in the elderly and in those undergoing elective surgery. The poor renal function association with electrolyte disturbances may affect the elimination of several drugs the anaesthetist uses.

Emergency operations have additional risks. The time to assess a patient may be short and insufficient to return him to his best state. With a major internal haemorrhage from a ruptured spleen or aorta the priority is to stop the bleeding; resuscitation goes on in parallel but need not precede haemostasis.

Fatness produces respiratory impairment in the grossly obese (and increases the technical difficulties for the surgeon). In elective surgery weight reduction beforehand will help everyone. The converse problem of starvation also has its hazards. The most striking examples are in those who have not been able to eat because of oesophageal cancer. Preoperative nutritional support may help them to overcome the metabolic stresses they will encounter.

The alphabet could go on but perhaps it is wisest here to leave it to those more directly concerned.

WHEN AND WHERE SHOULD PATIENTS BE ASSESSED?

Traditionally patients are assessed by the houseman on the day of admission. Most anaesthetists now assess their own patients—the night before operation for inpatients and immediately before the operation for day cases. Both systems give problems. The houseman may not have the knowledge of specific anaesthetic problems. The anaesthetist may detect problems that need further investigation or treatment or both and yet he is under some pressure not to disrupt the planned schedule of operations.

With long delays in the admission of many patients an assessment at the time of deciding to perform the operation will miss major problems developing in the intervening months (and years). In such cases Burn[10] developed a preoperative assessment clinic where the anaesthetist sees the patients he is to anaesthetise two weeks later. Problems can be identified, investigations made, and treatment offered. Should the operation not be needed or needs delaying there is time still to arrange another admission.

VALUE OF PREOPERATIVE ASSESSMENT

So far I have dealt with the use of a preoperative visit to assess the problems likely to be met with by the anaesthetist in dealing with the patient. There is another gain. One of my teachers of anaesthesia referred to herself as the "patient's friend." It is still surprising how many patients ask what is to be done to them—and why. Perhaps the anaesthetist, appearing late in the afternoon or evening, is less intimidating than the full surgical team, but information about the operation, anaesthetic, and likely postoperative treatment is usually accepted. Preoperative visiting should reassure both the anaesthetist and the patient.

REFERENCES

1. Harrison GG. Death attributable to anaesthesia. A 10-year survey (1967–76). *Br J Anaesth*, 1978;**50**:1041–6.
2. Tomkinson J, Turnbull A, Robson G, Cloake E, Adelstein AM, Weatherall J. *Report on confidential enquiries into maternal deaths in England and Wales.* London: HMSO, 1979.
3. Fisher M. Misery acquaints a man with strange bedfellows. *World Medicine* 1978;**14**:110–1.
4. American Society of Anaesthesiologists. New classification of physical status. *Anaesthesiology*, 1963;**24**:111.
5. Dripps RD, Lamont A, Eckenhoff JE. The role of anaesthesia in surgical mortality. *JAMA* 1961;**178**:261–6.
6. Goldman L, Caldera DL, Nussbaum SR, *et al.* Multifactorial index of cardiac risk in non-cardiac surgical procedures. *N Engl J Med* 1977;**297**:845–50.
7. Milledge JS, Nunn JF. Criteria of fitness for anaesthesia in patients with chronic obstructive lung disease. *Br Med J* 1975;iii:670–6.
8. Pugh RN, Murray-Lyon IM, Dawson JL, Pictroni MC, Williams R. Transection of the oesophagus for bleeding oesophageal varices. *Br J Surg* 1973;**60**:646–9.
9. Alberti KGMM, Thomas DJB. The management of diabetes during surgery. *Br J Anaesth* 1979;**51**:693–710.
10. Burn JMB. Preoperative anaesthetic assessment clinic. *Lancet* 1974;ii:886–8.

Care of the unconscious

JEAN M HORTON

Normal conscious behaviour means awareness of self and the environment and depends on intact brain function.[1] Changes in the level of consciousness reflect an abnormal function of the brain. The degree, depth, and duration of altered consciousness may vary from drowsiness to brain death, and "coma" or unconsciousness is best defined as an inability to obey commands, utter recognisable words, or open the eyes.[2]

Pathological conditions associated with this state are brain injury from trauma; cerebrovascular accidents; hypoxia; hypotension (low perfusion states); uncontrolled epilepsy; and disorders of metabolism, such as hepatic and renal failure and drug overdose.

As well as managing the primary cause of the coma, energetic treatment is needed to prevent the complications of unconsciousness, the most serious of which are hypoxia and hypotension.

All unconscious patients run the risk of an obstructed airway from the tongue falling back into the oropharynx. The inability to cough or swallow leads to an accumulation of secretions in the mouth, pharynx, trachea, and bronchi. Vomit and regurgitated gastric contents may be inhaled giving rise to the acid-aspiration (Mendelson's) syndrome in the lungs. The already damaged brain cannot withstand any further insults that may occur from inadequate cerebral oxygenation and perfusion due to a low arterial Po^2 or low blood pressure.[3]

The unconscious patient may need total care for days, weeks, or months, the problems being those of maintaining vital functions (adequate ventilation, circulation, and nutrition) and general nursing care.

Anaesthesia is a pharmacologically induced state of unconsciousness, and the well-trained anaesthetists of today, with their skill in care of the airway, endotracheal intubation, intravenous cannulation, ventilator management, and knowledge of applied pharmacology and respiratory physiology, are particularly able to care for these patients. The skills and lessons learnt in the operating theatre have enabled them to take part in the development, organisation, and management of patients in immediate care schemes and intensive treatment units and to teach these skills to other doctors, nurses, paramedical staff, and ambulance men.

IMMEDIATE MANAGEMENT

As soon as an unconscious patient is seen it is vital to establish and maintain a clear airway, adequate oxygenation, and alveolar ventilation, and satisfactory cardiovascular function is needed to maintain the cerebral perfusion pressure.

The mouth and pharynx should be cleared of any debris, dentures, blood, and vomit and the patient turned into the semiprone position (fig), so that the tongue can fall forwards, and the lower jaw should be pulled forward by placing the hands under the angle of the mandible. This manoeuvre should be performed with great care if there is any suspicion of a neck injury. An oropharyngeal airway of the Guedel type can then be inserted, but the patient may resist and vomiting, coughing, and bleeding be provoked.

A nasopharyngeal airway is an alternative and has the advantage of being tolerated at much lighter levels of consciousness, can be inserted into a patient whose jaw is tightly clenched, and provides a ready passage

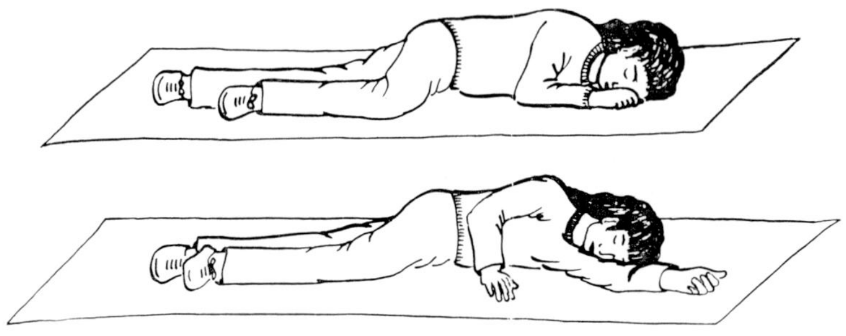

Two semiprone positions for unconscious patients.

for a suction catheter.[4] With this type of airway protection, which is not foolproof, the patient must be kept under very close observation. If these measures are not adequate because of an inefficient cough reflex or obvious respiratory failure a cuffed endotracheal tube should be passed. The aid of a short-acting neuromuscular blocker, such as suxamethonium, may be needed if there is much masseteric or laryngeal spasm, and cricoid pressure may help to prevent the regurgitation of stomach contents.

Endotracheal intubation is not always easy in the unconscious patient and should be performed only by competent, trained people. Persistent attempts at intubation can provoke bleeding and exacerbate hypoxia, and unrecognised oesophageal intubation can be disastrous. An alternative to endotracheal intubation is the cuffed oesophageal obturator airway, which does not require the use of a laryngoscope for its passage and prevents the regurgitation of vomit and inflation of the stomach with air.[5] There may be occasions during the initial management of an unconscious patient when relief of complete airway obstruction is impossible, and urgent tracheotomy or cricothyrotomy may be necessary. As a first-aid measure a wide bore (2-3 mm) needle can be passed through the cricothyroid membrane and enough oxygen can be given to sustain life. When a clear airway has been established 100% oxygen should be administered until the appropriate oxygen requirements can be determined from the results of arterial blood gas analysis.

All unconscious patients should have a gastric tube passed through the nose unless there is a head injury with fractures of the base of the skull or frontal sinuses, when the oral route is preferred. The gastric tube provides a route for oral feeding and aspiration of unabsorbed stomach contents. Should there be problems with the passage of the tube, an anaesthetist can often help by passing it through a long endotracheal tube that has been gently inserted into the oesophagus.

Before a definitive assessment of the unconscious patient is made or he is moved from the scene of an accident or incident, or from one department to another within a hospital or transferred to another hospital, the airway must be protected, hypotension corrected, and the patient accompanied by a trained escort, who is equipped with appropriate resuscitation and suction apparatus.

ASSESSMENT AND ROUTINE OBSERVATIONS

The condition of the unconscious patient may be changing all the time and so continuous observation is essential, since signs of deterioration will call for urgent action. The following observations should be made when the patient is first seen and then at least half-hourly and recorded on an appropriate chart, which is designed to be easily understood by medical and nursing staff and should show trends from which subsequent changes can be evaluated.

Conscious level

An alteration in the conscious level will precede all other changes in the vital and neurological signs.[6] The level of consciousness should be established as soon as possible, and an accurate description of behaviour is needed. A useful method of assessment is the Glasgow coma scale,[7] which is clear and informative and avoids the use of confusing terms such as semi-conscious, stupor, or semicomatose. It depends on the observation and recording of the response to three separate aspects of behaviour, which are eye opening, verbal responses, and the motor response to a verbal command or painful stimulus. The observer must be aware that the conscious level can remain influenced by hypoxia, sedatives, general anaesthesia, alcohol,[8] and metabolic problems.

Vital signs

The pulse rate and rhythm, systolic and diastolic blood pressure, pulse pressure, respiratory rate and pattern, and temperature must all be recorded.

A slow pulse, a rise in blood pressure, and slowing of respiration leading to periodic respiration and apnoea are signs of cerebral compression. A rising pulse and falling blood pressure are associated with haemorrhage and septic shock, and a rising pulse and blood pressure and rapid shallow respirations with hypoxia.

Focal neurological signs

Pupils—The pupils should be examined with a good light. The incidence of pupillary abnormalities in comatose patients is high, and careful attention should be given to the size, shape, and reaction to light.

Movement of the limbs—If localised brain damage is suspected additional assessment of the movement of each limb is needed in response to a verbal command or painful stimulus.

LONG-TERM CARE

Airway and ventilation

A clear airway and adequate alveolar ventilation, having been established, must be maintained. Auscultation of the chest, a chest radiograph, and determination of arterial blood gases should be performed daily. The PaO^2 should not be allowed to fall below 9·5 kPa (70 mm Hg) and an accurate prescription of a supplemental oxygen given if necessary using high air flow oxygen entrainment devices. When oxygen is administered care should be taken not to allow the PaO^2 to arise above 20 kPa (150 mm Hg), so as to avoid oxygen toxicity. The $PaCO^2$ should lie within the normal range of 4·5-6 kPa (34-46 mm Hg) except when therapeutic hyperventilation is needed for the management of cerebral oedema, when the $PaCO^2$ should not be allowed to fall below 3·3 kPa (25 mm Hg). Controlled mechanical ventilation of the lungs may be necessary in cases of respiratory failure or severe head injuries and other intracranial problems.

Prolonged airway care will be necessary in those patients where lengthy coma is anticipated and until they can care for their own airway. In the choice of method the advantages of intubation or tracheostomy must be weighed against the risks and the facilities available. The safe period of endotracheal intubation is not defined, but it would appear to be about seven days.[9] The cuffs on the endotracheal and tracheostomy tubes should be of the low-pressure type and the inspired air and oxygen humidified.

Regular tracheobronchial suction will be needed to remove secretions, and the patient should be turned from side to side every two hours to encourage drainage from all lobes of the lungs. Physiotherapists can be of immense service and should visit the patients at least twice a day, trying to coincide with turning periods. They should also carry out vibration and rib springing of the chest wall except when there are fractured ribs, when gentle percussion will suffice. If controlled ventilation is in use some physiotherapists find that a period of manual hyperventilation helps to express secretions into the tracheobronchial tree. Bronchoscopy should rarely be necessary and is best performed with a fibreoptic instrument.

Cardiovascular function

The importance of maintaining an adequate cerebral perfusion pressure has already been emphasised, and the systolic blood pressure should not be allowed to fall below 80-90 mm Hg. Also, it is now known that arterial hypertension in the presence of brain damage may lead to increased formation of cerebral oedema, so systolic blood pressures above 160 mm Hg should be avoided. The hypertension may be due to hypoxia, pain, a full bladder, restlessness, or an expanding brain lesion that must be excluded before prescribing sedation, analgesics, and antihypertensive treatment to maintain reasonable control of the blood pressure. A small dose of intravenous chlorpromazine 2·5-5 mg will often both sedate and lower blood pressure, but occasionally more powerful hypotensive drugs are needed, such as hydrallazine 5-10 mg and labetalol 10-20 mg.

Fluid and electrolyte balance

Severe brain damage may produce complicated metabolic and hormonal upsets, and a careful watch must be kept on the concentrations of plasma sodium, potassium, bicarbonate, urea, and creatinine, and osmolarity by daily estimation, which together with fluid balance intake and output charts will avoid the dangers of under- or over-hydration. An intravenous fluid regimen may be necessary, but in patients with cerebral oedema it is wise to restrict fluid maintenance to not more than 65-75% of normal.

Nutrition and feeding

As previously mentioned, all unconscious patients should have a gastric tube passed through the nose unless there is a risk of cerebrospinal fluid rhinorrhoea. The tube should be aspirated every two hours and be retained until the swallowing reflex returns. Oral fluids are not needed for the first 12 hours and then, provided that bowel sounds are present, an oral feeding regimen may be used. The quantity of feed may have to be adjusted according to the patient's total fluid requirements and balanced against any intravenous fluids being given. The use of fine bore nasogastric tubes and continuous oral feeding is not recommended in unconscious patients who have absent or inadequate gag reflexes and whose airways are not protected by cuffed endotracheal or tracheostomy tubes, as there is a danger of regurgitation of feeds and aspiration pneumonia. If oral feeds are not tolerated intravenous feeding may be necessary, and an anaesthetist may be asked to insert a central venous catheter for this purpose.

A serious complication of brain injury and coma which may upset nutrition and electrolyte and fluid balance is gastrointestinal bleeding. This may be due to "stress," steroids, or the presence of the nasogastric tube. If the patient is receiving steroids oral aluminium hydroxide and an H_2-receptor blocking agent may prevent this complication.[10]

Sedation and analgesics

Unconscious patients pass through a period of restless, disorganised behaviour before they regain a normal conscious level. This may be useful as the lungs and limbs are exercised, but the restlessness can be due to hypoxia, a full bladder, or pain. Provided that cerebral compression has been excluded sedation may be given, promazine 25-50 mg or chlorpromazine 25-50 mg being the most useful. For pain potent narcotic analgesics that cause respiratory depression should be avoided, and dihydrocodeine tartrate 30-60 mg or codeine phosphate 30-60 mg may be given. Local anaesthetic nerve blocks can also be used to reduce pain from, for example, fractured ribs or a fractured femur.

General nursing care

Eyes—Some unconscious patients lie with their eyes open and have an inefficient corneal reflex, which leaves the cornea exposed and may lead to keratitis and corneal ulcers. The eyes should be swabbed every two hours with physiological saline to remove discharge and debris. Artificial tears (0·3% hypromellose drops) should be instilled every two hours and the eyes kept shut with small pieces of strapping or a stitch through the upper lid, the threads being secured to the cheek by strapping. Should infection occur chloromycetin ointment is recommended.

Mouth care—Dentures should have been removed. There is a risk of parotitis if the mouth is not kept clean, and it should be swabbed every two hours with sodium bicarbonate followed by glycerin and thymol mouth wash. If the mouth is very dirty and crusted cleaning with hydrogen peroxide is useful. Yellow paraffin applied to the lips prevents angular stomatitis.

Bladder—Incontinence and wet beds predispose to bed sores. Men who are seriously ill will need catheterising for five to seven days. A catheter may then usually be replaced by Paul's tubing taped around the penis and the urine collected in a bottle. Women will need to be catheterised, but for a short term may lie on incontinence pads.

Bowels—Immobility and lack of dietary fibre result in constipation. Sennoside or danthron can be given down the gastric tube daily to stimulate the bowel and soften the stools. Enemas or manual evacuation every third day may be necessary. There is a risk of diarrhoea from infection, antibiotics, hyperosmolar feeds, bolus feeding, and attempting to institute a full feeding regimen too quickly. The diarrhoea can be checked with kaolin and by stopping the feeds.

Skin and pressure areas—To avoid pressure necrosis of the skin the patients should be kept clean and dry. They should be turned every two hours and washed once a day. Sheepskins are useful for the patient to lie on and as heel pads.

Limbs—The limbs should be taken through a range of active assisted movement daily by the physiotherapist to prevent contractures.

Temperature control—Hyperpyrexia may be due to several factors—infections of the respiratory tract, urinary tract, or wounds; drug reactions; or damage to the hypothalamic temperature-regulating centre. The temperature should be kept below 38°C and the fever treated by cooling the patient with a fan and a wet sheet. Chlorpromazine 25-50 mg every six hours and aspirin suppositories may be necessary as well as appropriate antibiotics.

Epilepsy—Convulsions may occur as a result of brain damage. It is important, however, to be cautious about giving immediate large doses of anticonvulsants that will depress the conscious level and make serial observations difficult. The development of severe epilepsy is serious. The consensus of opinion is that an intravenous injection of diazepam or clonazepam is the most effective way of treating this. Also chlormethiazole can be given by intravenous infusion, as can thiopentone. Paraldehyde is useful when there are no veins, and in intractable cases it may be necessary to paralyse and ventilate the patient. In all cases it is important to give maintenance doses of phenytoin to produce therapeutic blood concentrations.

CONCLUSION

A successful outcome for patients with recoverable causes of coma requires a consistently high standard of care and close co-operation among anaesthetists, clinicians, nursing staff, physiotherapists, and ambulance personnel. The importance of information and counselling for the relatives should not be forgotten.

REFERENCES

[1] Plum F, Posner JB. The pathological physiology of signs and symptoms of coma. In: *The diagnosis of stupor and coma*. Philadelphia: FA Davis Company, 1972:1–63.

[2] Jennett B, Teasdale G. Aspects of coma after severe head injury. *Lancet* 1977; i:878–81.

[3] Price DJE, Murray A. Influence of hypoxia and hypotension on recovery from head injury. *Injury*, 1972;**3**:218–24.

4 Zorab JSM, Baskett PJE. *Immediate care*. London, Philadelphia, Toronto: WB Saunders, 1977:10–22.
5 Harries MC. Mechanical aids to ventilation for use in the field. *Br Med J* 1979;ii:426–8.
6 Troupp H. Neurological problems in trauma deployment of resources. In: Walker WF, Taylor DEM, eds. *Intensive care*. Edinburgh: Churchill Livingstone, 1975:199–206.
7 Teasdale G, Jennett B, Assessment of coma and impaired consciousness, a practical scale. *Lancet*, 1974;ii:81–4.
8 Galbraith S, Murray WR, Patel AR, Knill-Jones R. The relationship between alcohol and head injury and its effect on the conscious level. *Br J Surg* 1976;**63**:128–30.
9 Aass AS. Complications to tracheostomy and long term intubation. A follow up study. *Acta Anaesthesiol Scand* 1975;**19**:127–33.
10 Burland WL, Parr SN. Experiences with cimetidine in the treatment of seriously ill patients. In: Burland WL, Simkins MA, eds. *Proceedings of the Second International Symposium on Histamine H_2-Receptor Antagonists*. Amsterdam, Oxford: Excerpta Medica, 1977:345–55.

Implications of day-case surgery and anaesthesia

T W OGG

In 1977 hospital day-case surgical procedures performed in England numbered 536 893, mainly in the specialties of urology, gynaecology, orthopaedics, and general surgery. Outpatient surgery was especially common in the larger regions—namely, Mersey, W Midlands, North-west, and Trent.

By definition day-case surgery is surgery performed on an outpatient basis with patients being admitted and discharged between 8 30 am and 5 pm. Ideally, surgery needing general anaesthesia should be undertaken during morning operating sessions.

British doctors are aware of the long NHS surgical waiting lists and of the need to increase efficiency and make financial savings within the expensive hospital service. Indeed, the Department of Health's planning guidelines for 1977-8 emphasised the need for the development of more day-surgery facilities.

In 1908 Nicoll operated successfully on 2392 children as outpatients in Glasgow.[1] Since then the work of several day-case units has been described.[2-4] The advantages and disadvantages of day surgery are outlined in the table.

Advantages and disadvantages of day-case surgery

Advantages	Disadvantages
Patients like day-case surgery	A second-rate service?
Ideal for children	Patient selection
Waiting lists decrease	Suitability of anaesthetic techniques
Infection rates decrease	Postoperative minor sequelae
Economic benefits	Medicolegal implications
Easy nursing staff recruitment	
Community services concerned	

Several questions must be answered before establishing a programme of day-case surgery: (1) Where will the surgery be performed? (2) Which surgical procedures can safely be undertaken? (3) Where, when, and by whom will the day cases be medically assessed? (4) Are modern general anaesthetic techniques satisfactory for outpatient work? (5) What will happen to these outpatients once discharged from hospital? (6) Will the general practitioner and community nursing services be able to cope?

ORGANISATION

Day surgery is an organisational exercise affecting the patient, medical records department, laboratories, hospital specialists, community services, and ambulance drivers. Ideally, a separate day-case unit should be established. A 10 to 12-bed unit will satisfy the needs of most British district general hospitals, and it need not be too expensive.[5] If senior hospital personnel are to participate in day-case surgery then the operating lists should be of suitable size to fill an operating session.

Patients scheduled for surgery should be issued with clear written and verbal instructions at their first surgical outpatient appointment. In every case the patient's general practitioner should be contacted for his advice on the suitability, both medical and social, of his patient attending for outpatient surgery.

An important factor is the availability of sufficient nursing staff for day-case units. The work entails a five-day week with no evenings or weekend duties. The advantages for the married nurse are obvious.

PREOPERATIVE ASPECTS

Where, when, and by whom should these patients be medically assessed? The general practitioner can play a major part in the preoperative medical assessment. Essentially healthy patients with good home conditions should be selected. Some day units impose an upper age limit of 65 years.

Before surgery these patients may be medically assessed in the surgical outpatient clinic, a preoperative anaesthetic clinic, or in the day unit on the day of operation by an experienced anaesthetist. All patients will have been instructed in advance to take nothing by mouth from the midnight before surgery. They will also have received advice not to take alcohol, return to work, or drive any vehicle or machinery for 24 hours after general anaesthesia. Ideally, all patients should be accompanied home by a responsible adult.

A preoperative assessment questionnaire has been used to assess 200 day cases.[6] The results showed a high incidence, almost 50%, of preexisting medical conditions and a drug history in 59% of cases. Great care should be taken in selecting these patients for day-case surgery.

Surgeons need not confine themselves to treating simple lumps and bumps. A few of the successful conditions operated on as day cases are the vaginal termination of pregnancy, cytoscopy, vasectomy, inguinal herniorrhaphy, varicose vein stripping, and surgery on the hand.

INTRAOPERATIVE ASPECTS

The challenge of outpatient anaesthesia for the anaesthetist is to produce a "street-fit" patient with few complications as soon as possible after the surgical procedure. The prerequisites of good day-case anaesthesia are a swift, safe induction with good intraoperative conditions, rapid recovery, and minimal postoperative morbidity.

Premedication is often omitted. Oral lorazepam 2 mg has been given to outpatients,[7] but its prolonged duration of action makes it unsuitable for patients returning home within eight hours of premedication. Furthermore, the routine use of the anticholinergic drugs, such as atropine and hyoscine, before minor surgery appears unnecessary.[8]

Which anaesthetic induction agent should be used? The popular thiobarbiturate, thiopentone, is inappropriate for day-case anaesthesia because of its slow metabolism and elimination from the body. Anaesthetists have therefore turned to methohexitone, propanidid, alphadolone alphaxalone (Althesin), and etomidate in recent years. Unfortunately, each of these agents has well-documented side effects. These include histamine release, thrombophlebitis, pain on injection, cardiovascular depression, involuntary muscle movements, and anaphylactic reactions. The fact is that the ideal anaesthetic induction agent, free from these undesirable side effects, has yet to be marketed.

In British hospitals the inhalational anaesthetic agent of choice for outpatients is halothane. A high incidence of postoperative sequelae, however, has been recorded after general anaesthesia with this agent.[9] An alternative may be the fluorinated ether, enflurane.[10] This inhalational anaesthetic agent gives a pleasant, safe induction with minimal cardiovascular depression and swift recovery.

Most anaesthetists will consider that their own day-case anaesthetic techniques are quite sufficient despite the pharmacological points already mentioned. More research is needed before the ideal outpatient anaesthetic of choice is found. Indeed, many surgical procedures may be satisfactorily performed under local analgesic. Some of these regional techniques include intravenous analgesia (Biers block) for limb surgery, digital nerve blocks for the wedge resection of toe-nails, and caudal analgesia for circumcision and anal procedures.

The use of muscle relaxants for outpatient operations is not without its problems. The common short-acting depolarising muscle relaxant, suxamethonium, is known to produce an appreciable incidence of vague muscle pains if early ambulation after surgery is encouraged. Small doses of non-depolarising relaxants, if given before suxamethonium, reduce but do not eliminate these muscle pains.

After fentanyl and methohexitone[11] it has been my practice in Cambridge to avoid inhalational anaesthetic agents for outpatients presenting for vaginal termination of pregnancy. For a woman weighing 70 kg I administer fentanyl 100 μg intravenously five minutes before surgery. This is followed by an induction dose of althesin 0·7 μl/kg. Anaesthesia is maintained with supplements of althesin 0·35 μl/kg as required while the patient breathes spontaneously room air or 100% oxygen. In 500 outpatients this technique has produced good operating conditions with swift recovery and minimal postoperative sequelae. This total intravenous approach to anaesthesia also eliminates the hazards of operating theatre pollution by inhalational anaesthetic gases.

When faced with dental outpatients needing 30 minutes of general anaesthesia how does one proceed? In my own dental practice I rarely use nasal endotracheal intubation. Using fentanyl and althesin as outlined above I pass a nasopharyngeal tube and pack the oropharynx with a Bristol oral V-pack. This technique is currently being investigated.

Recently the use of the non-specific respiratory stimulant doxapram[12] has been described for outpatient urological cases. This drug appears to ensure the swift, safe return to consciousness after simple anaesthesia.

POSTOPERATIVE ASPECTS

In one series 44·5% of patients undergoing day surgery had post-operative symptoms attributable to the general anaesthesia.[13] One hundred day cases have been assessed during the postoperative period[14] to discover what happened to them once they left the hospital confines. An appreciable morbidity was recorded—for instance, nausea, vomiting, dizziness, and drowsiness. Of these patients, 30% had disregarded medical advice and journeyed home unaccompanied while 9% of car owners had driven themselves home.

These findings have important medicolegal implications. Car owners should be instructed not to drive for 24 hours after general anaesthesia or at the very least until after they have had a good night's sleep. Much research has detailed the adverse effects of alcohol and driving. Apart from laboratory studies, surprisingly few reports have outlined the dangers of general anaesthesia and impaired driving ability.

The early discharge of day cases from hospital does not impose an intolerable work load on general practitioners. It is the community nursing services which become most concerned with these patients. All day-case units should have easy access to hospital inpatient beds if the occasional patient has to be admitted. Any problems that may arise once the patient returns home should immediately be notified to the surgeon or anaesthetist concerned with the case.

Why do patients often disregard medical advice in the immediate postoperative period? Recently it has been found that patients suffer from considerable memory impairment for new facts after simple general anaesthesia.[15] Further research is in progress to determine which anaesthetic agents produce the least disturbance of memory. At present, anaesthetists have no single, simple, reliable practical test of recovery for assessing patient street-fitness after general anaesthesia.

Finally, patients will often need postoperative analgesia once they return home. Many will be satisfactorily treated with simple oral analgesics — for instance, paracetamol and dextropropoxyphene

(Distalgesic). On occasion, however, an opiate needs to be prescribed. An interesting drug is buprenorphine, a synthetic, non-addictive opiate with a prolonged action, which can be administered sublingually.

Postoperative pain relief may also be treated by several local analgesic techniques. Caudal analgesia with bupivacaine 0·5% or 0·25% solution has a definite place after painful anal or penile surgery.

CONCLUSIONS

If surgical waiting lists continue to increase and financial allocations to the NHS decrease then doctors will have to consider suitable alternatives to present-day practices. Day-case surgery is one method of reducing these large waiting lists. There are many problem areas, but they are not insurmountable. The establishment of more day-case units should be encouraged and the organisation of these units must be first class. The following guidelines are essential for safe day-case surgical and anaesthetic practice.

(1) Day-case surgery should not be a second-class service.
(2) Separate day units should be established.
(3) Senior hospital staff must participate.
(4) Efficient preoperative screening is essential.
(5) More research into simple anaesthetic techniques should be performed.
(6) The recovery period must have a low morbidity.
(7) Co-operation among the patient, hospital consultants, general practitioner, and community nursing services is essential for the project to succeed.

REFERENCES

1 Nicoll JH. Surgery of infancy. *Br Med J* 1909;ii:753.
2 Stephens FO, Dudley HAF. An organisation for outpatient surgery. *Lancet* 1961;i:1042–4.
3 Berrill TH. A year in the life of a surgical day unit. *Br Med J* 1972;iv:348–9.
4 Rainey JB, Ruckley CV. Work of a day-bed unit 1972–8. *Br Med J* 1979;ii: 714–7.
5 Calnan J, Martin P. Development and practice of an autonomous minor surgery unit in a general hospital. *Br Med J* 1971;iv:92–6.
6 Ogg TW. Assessment of preoperative cases. *Br Med J* 1976;i:82–3.
7 Loach A, Fisher A. Lorazepam as a premedicant for day-case surgery: an assessment. *Anaesthesia* 1975;**30**:545–9.
8 Mirakhur RK, Dundee JW, Connolly JDR. Studies of drugs given before anaesthesia. XVII Anticholinergic premedicants. *Br J Anaeths* 1979;**51**: 339–45.
9 Smith BL, Young PW. Day stay anaesthesia: a follow-up of day patients undergoing dental operations under general anaesthesia with tracheal intubation. *Anaesthesia* 1976;**31**:181–9.
10 Black GW, Johnston HML, Scott MG. Clinical impressions of enflurane. *Br J Anaesth* 1977;**49**:875–80.
11 Goroszeniuk T, Whitwam JG, Morgan M. Use of methohexitone, fentanyl and nitrous oxide for short surgical procedures. *Anasethesia* 1977;**32**:209–11.

[12] Riddell PL, Robertson GS. Use of doxapram as an arousal agent in outpatient general anaesthesia. *Br J Anaesth* 1978;**50**:921–4.
[13] Fahy A, Marshall M. Postanaesthetic morbidity in outpatients. *Br J Anaesth* 1969;**41**:433–7.
[17] Ogg TW. An assessment of postoperative outpatient cases. *Br Med J* 1972;iv: 573–6.
[15] Ogg TW, Fischer HBJ, Bethune DW, Collis JM. Day case anaesthesia and memory. *Anaesthesia* 1979;**34**:784–9.

Postoperative care

A A SPENCE

In earlier times survival from the physiological challenge of a surgical operation was so unpredictable that the lesser risks to life (let alone the discomfort) of the postoperative period were not considered important. Today, patients presenting for routine elective surgery expect to survive and, for the population as a whole, this can be guaranteed only if the quality of postoperative care is equal to that available within the operating room itself.

RESPIRATORY PROBLEMS

The traditional routine of the surgical ward is surprisingly ill suited to the acute demands that may occur in the immediate postoperative period (1–4 hours); thus typically the recovery room serves to concentrate medical and nursing attention for all the patients in an entire operating suite, the likely case load determining the size of the facility. As a rule one nurse is required for every four patients, and there must be ready access from the theatres so that surgeons and anaesthetists can attend their patient if necessary. There is a variety of need to which the staff and equipment must be suited. Some patients will be admitted before their protective reflexes have returned, and they are at risk from the several causes of airway obstruction, including regurgitation of gastric contents. Even when the patient has wakened the defence against accidental aspiration may be obtunded for several hours, particularly in the elderly and patients of any age in whom neuromuscular blocking drugs, such as tubocurarine, have not been antagonised adequately. If this last problem is suspected or if there are reasons to suspect ventilatory inadequacy because of the type of incision or the preoperative respiratory state of the patient artificial ventilation of the lungs may be continued or reinstituted.

After many types of anaesthesia and surgery there will be an abnormally large right-to-left shunt of the pulmonary blood flow resulting in arterial hypoxaemia when the patient breathes air.[1] For example, in a healthy patient who has undergone upper abdominal surgery the arterial oxygen tension (Pao_2) may be reduced by about 3 kPa (22·5 mm Hg). This problem is exaggerated if the cardiac output (pulmonary blood flow) is abnormally low. In routine cases these events are expected, and the administration of 30–40% oxygen from a suitable mask will correct the deficiency. If there is pre-existing lung disease affecting Pao_2 the effect of surgery is additive. Thus in addition to giving oxygen Pao_2 should be measured to ensure that blood oxygenation is adequate. While it is not possible to consider here the various conditions that may present, as a general rule Pao_2 less than 8 kPa (60 mm Hg) in the immediate postoperative period is undesirable and may necessitate other measures, such as artificial ventilation of the lungs.

CARDIOVASCULAR PROBLEMS

Second in importance to respiratory care in the recovery room is the need to monitor the cardiovascular system and correct deficiencies. A basic requirement is the regular checking of arterial pressure and pulse rate every 15–20 minutes. In patients with heart disease and all who have or are likely to have serious disturbances of rhythm the ECG must be monitored, typically with an oscilloscope display, although chart-recording facilities may be required. Other indices of circulatory adequacy of deterioration include central venous pressure measurement, urine output, and careful charting of blood and other fluid losses from drainage tubes etc.

Monitoring and care of the circulation is particularly important in patients who have undergone cardiac surgery including extracorporeal bypass and those in whom arterial hypotension has been induced deliberately to improve operating conditions or reduce blood loss (in middle ear or pelvic surgery, for example). In such cases direct monitoring and display of the arterial and central venous pressure, measurement of cardiac output and body temperature, and the storage or display of such information may place special demands on both training and space in the recovery room.

LACK OF PAIN RELIEF

It is the scandal of modern surgery that a large proportion of patients suffer severe pain in the postoperative period. While there is no lack of feasible methods of pain relief there is a surprising reluctance to use them. The blame for this must be shared by surgeons and nurses but particularly by anaesthetists, whose special profession is the relief of pain.

In the vast majority of cases a prescription is written for a narcotic analgesic to be administered by intramuscular injection "as required," often with some qualification as to the minimum interval between injections. While this practice may presuppose timely treatment for each patient on the part of the nursing staff, day and night, even casual consideration of the normal administrative arrangements for the use of narcotics by nurses in hospital, and of the many other calls on the nurses' time, indicates that such assumptions are unwarranted.

It must be stated frankly that the alternatives are either more expensive or time consuming, or both.

The intravenous "titration" of narcotics against the patient's pain has established superiority to the intramuscular route. Contemporary understanding of opiate receptors in the central nervous system explains why relatively small doses of these drugs given intravenously provide better relief with a comparable duration of action.

Recent developments include programmed automatic syringe systems that allow safe intravenous administration of a narcotic by the patient himself. Having the means of analgesia at hand is popular with patients and may reduce the anxiety associated with pain to the extent that drug requirements are less and the quality of relief better than in conventional practice. Other self-administered methods include inhalation analgesia (premixed 50% nitrous oxide in oxygen (Entonox) or trichloroethylene or methoxyflurane in air), which have been very successful in clinical trials. The benefits of transcutaneous electrical stimulation are by no means certain.

Perhaps the most effective method of analgesia, because in most cases the relief is total, is nerve blockade by local anaesthetic; there are various methods depending on the site of surgery. The most popular with anaesthetists is extradural nerve block, in which a catheter is passed through a needle inserted into the extradural space roughly in the midpoint of the range of nerve segments to be blocked—for instance, T5-T11 for a right upper paramedian incision. The local anaesthetic solution is injected in a volume sufficient to block the required range of nerves and repeat injections are given after the early signs of returning discomfort; in a typical case in which bupivacaine 0·25–0·5% is used the injections may need to be repeated every two hours. Such blockade may be extended for several days if necessary, but the normal requirement is usually not more than 48 hours.

Intercostal nerve block in which a local anaesthetic solution is deposited around the intercostal nerve, usually at the posterior angle of the rib, when compared with extradural block has the advantage of a much longer duration, perhaps eight hours after a single injection, but there is no ease of access for repeat injection comparable with the extradural catheter. Intercostal injections carry the risk of inducing a pneumothorax, although in skilled hands this is unlikely. The method is particularly suitable for transverse incisions on one side of the body, such as the Kocher's incision for cholecystectomy. Nerve block techniques may be life-saving in protecting high-risk patients from pulmonary insufficiency associated with surgical pain in the postoperative period. They are technically demanding, however, and call for a high quality of supervision by both nurses and doctors. Extradural block may be associated with postural hypotension, particularly in patients whose circulatory volume is less than normal. A rare possibility is the risk of accidental subarachnoid injection of the local anaesthetic solution resulting in the need for artificial ventilation as an emergency. Such problems are rare, however, and in experienced hands are not an impediment to the use of these valuable methods.

RECOVERY ROOMS

Twenty years ago postoperative recovery rooms were virtually unknown in British hospitals. Doctors and nurses whose experience extends to that time have usually no difficulty in recalling the crises and occasional disasters that accompanied unattended airway obstruction, regurgitation and aspiration, ventilatory failure, or cardiac arrest in patients who had recently returned to the surgical ward from the operating theatre. Equally vivid are the recollections of fear in the young nurse detailed as a "special" nurse (usually behind the screens) for the high-risk postoperative patient.

Today the recovery room is an integral part of surgical practice and an essential component in progressive patient care. In several countries of the Western world, but particularly in Scandinavia, the concept has been extended to allow patients who have undergone major, routine surgery to receive the benefits of the more highly serviced recovery area in preference to the surgical ward for up to 24 hours. Such arrangements permit a logical deployment of nursing skills, particularly in times of staff shortages, and improve the quality of monitoring and record keeping. The direct benefit to the patient includes careful treatment of his pain: recovery room nurses have more time than those in the surgical ward to learn and practise the skills of intravenous or inhalation analgesia or to maintain nerve block analgesia by injection through a catheter.

The ideal is for the recovery room and the intensive care unit to be adjacent to allow medical support for the former in an emergency. Those with experience of this type of service, however, emphasise that the roles of the recovery area and of the intensive care unit are different and that only rarely should a patient need to be moved from one to the other. Thus a patient known to be suffering from septic shock or from severe chronic lung disease should be admitted to the intensive care unit, bypassing the recovery facilities.

There are early indications that 24-hour recovery facilities will become accepted in Britain over the next ten years; if this does happen it will constitute a major improvement in surgical care.

REFERENCE

[1] Spence AA. Postoperative pulmonary complications. In: Gray TC, Nunn JF, Utting JE, eds. *General anaesthesia*. 4th ed. Vol 1. London: Butterworth, 1980:591–608.

The anaesthetist in the accident and emergency service

PETER J F BASKETT

The basic training of the anaesthetist in the operating room is orientated around secure airway control, artificial ventilation, monitoring and support of the circulation, and the relief of acute pain. It is precisely these skills that are essential in managing the suddenly ill and seriously injured patients cared for by the accident and emergency services and departments (fig 1).

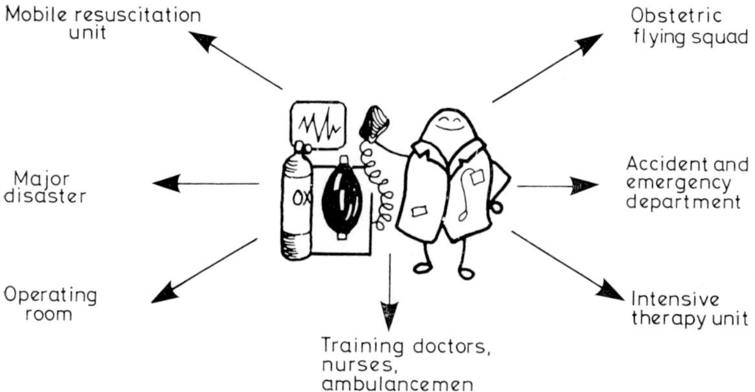

FIGURE 1—Roles of the anaesthetist.

PREHOSPITAL CARE

Increasing awareness in several countries of the world of the value of expert prehospital care has led to the development in Britain of schemes designed to bring skilled assessment and treatment to the patient on site and during transport to hospital. In certain rural areas general practitioners [1] have organised on-site immediate care schemes. Through training in hospital with anaesthetists in the anaesthetic rooms, operating theatres, and recovery rooms they have acquired the skills of intravenous cannulation and transfusion, airway control using endotracheal intubation, and reliable artificial ventilation with a self-inflating bag or mechanical resuscitator. In urban areas general-practitioner schemes are not so practical, and several centres [2,3] have now followed the United States practice of training selected ambulance personnel to a paramedical standard, which includes the practical skills mentioned above combined with a thorough knowledge and understanding of the systematic assessment and monitoring of the seriously ill patient.[4]

All of these paramedical schemes rely on anaesthetists for a large part of their training and, in several instances, the entire scheme has been masterminded and organised by anaesthetists working in collaboration with their colleagues in the accident and emergency department and in the ambulance service. There are now moves to improve the efficiency of the emergency side of the ambulance service in Britain by separating this part away from the routine transport service, thereby creating a top tier of highly trained men to concentrate on the patients requiring skilled emergency care. As this development is adopted by more and more centres, so anaesthetists will become increasingly concerned. It is important, however, that they do not confine their participation to training only. They should also work on site from time to time with the trainees in their own environment to appreciate the problems of attempting resuscitation away from the complex and organised surroundings of their hospital.

OBSTETRIC FLYING SQUAD

With improving antenatal care by general practitioners and obstetricians and the increasing trend towards hospital rather than domiciliary confinement, the need for obstetric flying squads has declined considerably in the past decade. The anaesthetist was an essential member of such squads, providing sedation for patients with eclampsia and resuscitation and anaesthesia for the serious postpartum haemorrhage. With the contracting requirement, many maternity units have abandoned the formal obstetric flying squad and prefer to treat the isolated case by arranging for the ambulance service to transport the anaesthetist and obstetrician and their essential equipment to the patient in a normal ambulance.

Thus the current emphasis is to provide resuscitation to ensure that the patient is fit for the journey to the local maternity hospital. Obstetric procedures outside hospital are kept to the bare minimum compatible with the patient's safety. Naturally, obstetric emergencies may be included in the facilities provided by any established mobile resuscitation unit for prehospital care in the area without appreciable extra organisation or use of resources.

ACCIDENT AND EMERGENCY DEPARTMENT

In most hospitals receiving emergency patients an anaesthetist in the accident and emergency department helps resuscitate seriously ill or injured patients brought into the department. The anaesthetist works as a member of the team with colleagues in the ambulance service, the accident and emergency staff, and, on occasion, other specialists relevant to the patient's illness or injury—for instance, neurosurgeons or thoracic surgeons, cardiologists, etc.

Several centres have appointed a consultant anaesthetist to the accident and emergency department on a part-time basis to help train the staff, both nursing and medical, and to advise on selection of resuscitation and life support equipment in the unit. This forges a link between the two specialties that is becoming stronger as more specialist consultants in accident and emergency work are appointed and the formal training of senior registrars in the specialty becomes established.

MAJOR DISASTER

Every area health authority has a responsibility to ensure that there is provision to cope with a major disaster. Part of the arrangements must include the dispatch of a mobile hospital team to the disaster site to organise triage and provide treatment of the casualties.[5] The anaesthetist is a member of this team and works alongside colleagues in surgery, nursing, and the ambulance service. They are indeed fortunate if they have had experience of working outside hospital with the emergency services in a mobile resuscitation unit designed to provide a day-to-day prehospital care service.

In some area plans the anaesthetist will act as the site medical officer, whose responsibility is to deploy the medical and paramedical teams in the most effective manner, liaise with the other emergency services, and communicate with the receiving hospitals. It is perhaps more important that the anaesthetist's special talents are reserved for the "hands on" resuscitation and treatment on site and in hospital rather than becoming concerned with administration and liaison, which can be performed by another, perhaps not so essential, doctor.

HOSPITAL CARDIAC ARREST SERVICE

Every district general hospital provides a team to attend to acute emergencies such as cardiorespiratory arrest occurring within the hospital precincts.[6] The anaesthetist is a vital member of this team, attending expertly in the emergency to artificial ventilation, endotracheal intubation, and the establishment of an intravenous route. The last may present considerable difficulty in the patient with circulatory standstill but can often be achieved by cannulation of the internal jugular or subclavian vein—techniques which are part of the anaesthetist's skills learnt in the operating theatre and intensive therapy unit and which have particular application in an emergency.

VARIETY OF PATIENTS

During their work in accident and emergency anaesthetists become concerned with a wide variety of patients due to their particular expertise (fig 2). In trauma they will make a particular contribution to patients with head, chest, and maxillofacial injuries where death is often caused by hypoxia and hypercarbia due to airway obstruction and inadequate pulmonary ventilation. The passage of an endotracheal tube in a patient with bizarre distortion of the normal anatomical features caused by a severe maxillofacial injury is extremely hazardous and calls

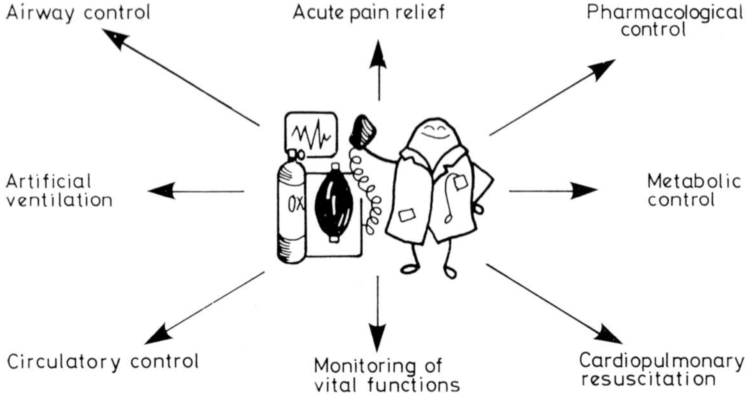

FIGURE 2—Expertise of the anaesthetist.

for special experience and skill in the technique. Control of ventilation in a patient with a chest injury complicated by pneumothorax and a ruptured bronchus requires a detailed knowledge of pulmonary mechanics and physiology and may require unique specialist skill in placing an endobronchial or double lumen tube to isolate the damaged lung. In certain isolated cases the two lungs may have to be ventilated separately using two different ventilators.

The prognosis of many patients with head injuries can be improved considerably by hyperventilation and, here again, the anaesthetists' expertise in techniques of artificial ventilation makes a major contribution. Hyperventilation reduces raised intracranial pressure, permitting an improvement in cerebral perfusion. Although the technique is usually applied by a mechanical ventilator in the intensive care unit, to be most effective it should really be instituted at the earliest possible opportunity during transport to hospital and in the accident and emergency department.

Any case of multiple trauma or acute surgical emergency, such as haematemesis or ruptured aortic aneurysm affecting massive blood loss, will need an anaesthetist to establish multiple reliable intravenous routes for blood replacement and to insert catheters to monitor the effects of resuscitation by arterial, central venous, and indirect left atrial pressures and cardiac output measurements.

Patients with trauma are normally in severe pain, which should be relieved, not only for humanitarian reasons but also because of the deleterious effects on tissue perfusion caused by the excessive secretion of catecholamines. The anaesthetist's detailed knowledge of analgesics and anaesthetics, their merits and their hazards, is of particular value in the early management of the trauma victim.

In accident and emergency the anaesthetist is not just concerned with surgical patients. Acute epiglottitis requires special intubating skills, and patients with an acute exacerbation of their chronic obstructive airways disease present conditions demanding accurate control of oxygenation and ventilation, which are part of the anaesthetist's basic training. Detailed knowledge of pharmacology of sedative, hypnotic, tranquillising, and narcotic agents combined with resuscitative expertise ensures that the anaesthetist has a place in the emergency management of patients suffering from drug overdose. These skills are also valuable in controlling patients with persistent convulsions. Many fatalities associated with acute myocardial infarction may be avoided by skilful arrhythmia control and early defibrillation in ventricular tachycardia and fibrillation. The anaesthetist, who is familiar with the pharmacological control of arrhythmias and with the defibrillator from his experience in the operating room, has a definite contribution to make as both teacher and participator.

CONCLUSION

The anaesthetist has a fundamental role in the immediate care of the critically ill and injured patient. Participation in the accident and emergency services at all stages is but one example of the breadth of skill that members of the specialty can offer in the care of patients, both inside and outside the operating room. The wide scope of interest and participation is an essential element in making the present-day work of an anaesthetist so varied and satisfying.

REFERENCES

[1] Easton K. Immediate care. In: Easton K, ed. *Rescue emergency care*. London: Heinemann, 1977:174.

[2] Chamberlain DA, White NM, Binning R, Parker WS, Kimber ER. Mobile coronary care provided by ambulance personnel. *Br Heart J* 1973;**35**:550.

[3] Baskett PJF, Diamond AW, Cochrane DF. Urban mobile resuscitation—training and service. *Br J Anaesth* 1976;**48**:377–85.

[7] Stewart RD. The training of paramedical personnel. In: Norman J, Moles M, eds. *Management of the injured patient*. London: MacMillan, 1978.

[5] Moles TM. Planning for major disasters. In: Norman J, Moles M, eds, *Management of the injured patient*. London: MacMillan, 1978.

[6] Marshall RD. A year of resuscitation. *Anaesthesia* 1966;**21**:86–91.

Intensive care

A B M TELFER

Since the advent of intensive care units in the 1960s anaesthetists have played a major part in their organisation and development. Although these units, especially in district hospitals, are usually multidisciplinary, they all cater for critically ill patients, most of whom need some form of life support, either respiratory, cardiac, or renal. Anaesthetists, by virtue of their training in the use of mechanical ventilation, patient monitoring, applied pharmacology, and the management of fluid balance, are particularly suited to this type of work, both from the clinical and administrative points of view.

One of the earliest publications on intensive care units[1] surveyed 17 units in Britain and reported that anaesthetists were in charge in seven of them, physicians in five, a surgeon in one, another was shared, and three were undecided who was in charge. Since that report was published 12 years have passed, and the frontiers of intensive care have expanded from the original units, which dealt solely with chronic respiratory failure—for example, in the Scandinavian poliomyelitis epidemic in 1952—to the present-day unit, which deals as much with circulatory and metabolic issues as it does with respiratory care.[2] Anaesthetists are in administrative charge of most units and also usually carry a considerable part of the clinical responsibility. Exactly how much depends very much on local arrangements and, perhaps most of all, on personalities. A prerequisite when in charge of an intensive care unit is an abundance of tact and diplomacy, since one is dealing with clinicians who have, to a greater or lesser degree, "handed over" their patient.

It may interest the general reader to have some idea of the nature of the wide variety of clinical problems dealt with in the present-day intensive care unit. The emphasis will vary in different locations, and for the purposes of this article I will exclude the special problems of the coronary care unit and of acute and chronic renal dialysis units, although many "general" intensive care units now have facilities for haemodialysis within the unit.

POSTOPERATIVE PATIENTS

Some older hospitals may have few and inadequate recovery facilities and therefore several patients have to be accommodated in the intensive care units after operation. They have mostly undergone emergency abdominal surgery—for example, for a leaking aortic aneurysm. Several admissions are also to be expected after elective surgery, usually those needing planned postoperative ventilatory support—for example, in patients with chronic respiratory disease who have undergone major surgery. In such patients the avoidance of hypoxia and the provision of adequate analgesia are of paramount importance in the immediate postoperative period. Techniques such as continuous epidural analgesia and the administration of intravenous narcotic analgesics, for instance, morphine, by continuous infusion pump[3] require a degree of supervision often to be found only in the intensive care unit.

Elective postoperative ventilation is also widely practised after cardiac surgery, especially when cardiopulmonary bypass has been undertaken and, again depending on the local circumstances, the intensive postoperative care that these patients require may be undertaken in the "general" intensive care unit or in a special unit devoted to the purpose. A strong case may be made for this latter arrangement, mainly on the grounds of infection. Thorp *et al*[4] recently reported an overall infection rate of 36% in one "general" intensive care unit—an incidence that would clearly not be acceptable to cardiac surgeons.

TRAUMA

Trauma continues to provide a steady flow of patients to intensive care units. Road traffic accidents, especially with motorcycles, are a common cause of serious injury. Although seat belts, when worn, have undoubtedly reduced the severity of injuries, these still occur with distressing frequency. Industrial accidents and serious assaults are also common, at least in certain localities.

Head injuries are included in this series and will not be further discussed here, except to say that when associated with a chest injury their already high mortality is further increased.

CLOSED CHEST INJURIES

Closed chest injuries are usually sustained in road traffic accidents, often associated with violent deceleration, which may initiate a dissecting aneurysm of the thoracic aorta, while contact with the steering wheel may cause appreciable myocardial trauma. More commonly, contusion of the lung with multiple fractures of the ribs occurs, and the physiological lesion is usually more important than the anatomical injury. The functional disturbance may vary from pain on deep breathing and coughing to frank respiratory failure needing mechanical ventilation. Particular attention must be paid to the presence of chronic obstructive airways disease, and especially to an acute exacerbation, when even a minor chest injury can precipitate respiratory failure. When the chest is "flailing" and paradoxical movement is present, intermittent positive-pressure ventilation (the so-called internal pneumatic stabilisation) is widely regarded as the treatment of choice; this may be needed for many days, and the full facilities of a respiratory intensive care unit are necessary.

Intensive care

The primary first aid at the scene of any accident and the immediate management in the hospital casualty department before admission to the unit may have a profound effect not only on subsequent recovery but on the quality of that recovery.

MULTIPLE INJURIES

Patients with multiple injuries present many problems, both immediate and delayed. There may, for example, be a need to anaesthetise for laparotomy a patient who has a major chest injury with serious loss of lung function. Pulmonary or coagulation problems may follow massive blood transfusion, or fat embolism may follow limb fractures.

All of these demand not only treatment but also the most careful monitoring. It is normal practice in major injuries to measure arterial blood pressure continuously[5] as well as central venous pressure and, when indicated, pulmonary artery and pulmonary artery wedge pressure, using a Swan-Ganz flow-directed catheter.

In addition, comparison of central and peripheral temperatures and estimation of hourly urine output give further information about organ blood flow, the maintenance of which is obviously of fundamental importance. This emphasis on monitoring, while important in all critically ill patients, is especially important in the injured. Their condition may change suddenly and dramatically, and early warning must be available if episodes of hypotension or hypoxia are to be avoided.

BURNS AND THERMAL INJURY

Inhalation injuries to the respiratory tract after a burning accident are associated with a high mortality—about 80%.[6] They may be present in the absence of obvious external burns and may be due to direct heat (from inhaling hot air) or to inhaling toxic and irritant smoke (especially if certain organic plastics are burning), and there may also be a blast effect if there has been an explosion in a confined space. In addition, particles of soot may be deposited in the respiratory tract, producing further local irritation, and the whole picture may be compounded by the effects of hypoxia.

Although they appear to be initially well, patients who may have been exposed to this type of trauma should always be admitted to hospital for observation since the toxic effects and physiological deterioration may appear later, and rapid intervention may be needed.

The fibreoptic bronchoscope has an important place in managing this type of lung injury, enabling particles of foreign material to be removed from the airways under direct vision.

DRUG OVERDOSE

Patients who have taken a sufficient quantity of a drug or drugs (and alcohol is such a drug) to render themselves unconscious face two dangers—the toxicological effects of the drug and the risks of lying unconscious with an unprotected and perhaps obstructed airway. Since vomiting or regurgitation is common in these cases, aspiration of gastric contents with pulmonary soiling is often a sequel. Hypothermia may also develop if the victim has been lying unattended for many hours, especially if drugs of the phenothiazine group have been taken.

Adequate monitoring and basic supportive treatment are all that are usually required. In relatively few cases is specific drug treatment indicated—for example, the cardiovascular effects of the tricyclic anti-depressants can be reversed with physostigmine, and naloxone will reverse the central respiratory depressant effect of narcotic overdosage (including Distalgesic overdose). Patients who have taken paracetamol should be transferred rapidly to hospital for the possible early administration of acetylcysteine to prevent subsequent liver damage.

Specific measures to accelerate excretion of drugs, such as peritoneal dialysis and haemodialysis, are now less often used than formerly, most workers believing that the safest method of excretion is by the patient's own urinary tract.

CHRONIC OBSTRUCTIVE AIRWAYS DISEASE

When acute infection, either bacterial or viral, is added to chronic obstructive airways disease, respiratory failure may soon follow. Many of these patients may be managed in medical wards with conservative measures, but some also require active intervention to remove bronchial secretions, and may need mechanical ventilation. Careful selection is needed and full discussion between the anaesthetist in the intensive care unit and the referring physician should take place before ventilation starts.

POLYNEURITIS

Polyneuritis may lead to respiratory failure which may last for many weeks in a patient who may be fully conscious, totally paralysed, and with a tracheostomy, and who therefore has a major problem in communication. On the other hand, the lungs themselves are unaffected, and therefore the actual process of mechanical ventilation should not be difficult.

TETANUS

Tetanus is not common in Britain, only 16 cases being notified in England and Wales in 1977. If the disease is suspected at all the patient should be referred to a hospital with an intensive care unit able to offer full facilities for respiratory care. The experience of one such unit, at Leeds, with 100 cases has been well documented by Edmondson and Flowers,[7] who reported a death rate of 10%.

CONVULSIVE STATES

The management of severe convulsions also comes within the remit of the intensive care unit. By definition a patient who is having convulsions is apnoeic and may therefore become severely hypoxic. This is most commonly seen in severe epilepsy, but convulsions from other causes may on occasions be severe enough to warrant admission to an intensive care unit. Such patients are managed by neuromuscular paralysis, mechanical ventilation, and appropriate anticonvulsant treatment. In at least one unit in Britain automatic administration of the anticonvulsant is achieved by using a feed-back signal from the electroencephalogram (Price, personal communication, 1979).

ACCIDENTAL HYPOTHERMIA

Hypothermia may occur as part of a disease, such as myxoedema, or result from lying immobile after trauma—for instance, a fractured femur in the elderly. It has already been mentioned under drug overdose. Its occurrence is often overlooked and only a high index of suspicion and a low reading thermometer may detect it. Such patients should be admitted to an intensive care unit for careful supervision of active rewarming.

NEAR-DROWNING

Immersion incidents with hypothermia and "near-drowning" occur both in fresh water inland areas and in coastal areas. In both cases the immediate first aid on the spot and the efficiency of transport to hospital have a major influence on the outcome. The delayed effects of near-drowning on the lungs, however, mean that, whenever possible, people who appear to have survived such an incident should be observed in hospital where full facilities for intensive care are available.[8]

There are many other conditions where respiratory support may be necessary—as in septic shock or when the lung lesion is secondary to other disease, for instance, pancreatitis, or is iatrogenic, for instance, overtransfusion. It should not be assumed, however, that the average patient in an intensive care unit has only a respiratory problem: cardiovascular, metabolic, renal, infective, and nutritional problems are all interlinked,[9] and attention to only one system is a sure recipe for disaster. In addition, there may be unique problems of communication with the patient and relatives, who may have to undergo a period of stress of a duration undreamt of 20 years ago.

Intensive care units are now a well-established and widely accepted part of the hospital scene. Over the years they have played a significant part in reducing mortality and morbidity in seriously ill patients by concentrating life-support equipment and skill and providing continuous monitoring of the patient's condition, both electronically and by the five (or six) senses of the attendant nurses. There is, however, an increasing need to know more about the patient and to know it continuously. Thus the future will see, in addition to developments in non-invasive monitoring, the increasing use of intravascular electrodes for continuous measurement of gas tensions and the more widespread use of pulmonary artery pressure measurements in assessing cardiac performance. The application of computing and data storage techniques to these and other variables enables derived values to be obtained immediately, thus allowing treatment to be based on a much greater appreciation of the extent of the physiological derangement.

Perhaps, above all, the intensive care unit sees no interdisciplinary barriers in patient management. It can, and does, call on all specialties in the hospital when required, from the bacteriologist to the radiologist, and the biochemist to the pharmacist, as well as physicians, surgeons, and anaesthetists. In this way, through the organisation of the unit, the full resources of the hospital are brought to bear on the most critically ill patients.

REFERENCES

[1] British Medical Association. *Planning Unit Report. No 1 Intensive Care.* London: BMA, 1967:15.
[2] Tinker J. The staffing and management of intensive therapy units. *Br J Hosp Med* 1976;**16**:399–406.
[3] Nayman J. Measurement and control of post-operative pain. *Ann R Coll Surg Eng* 1979;**61**:419–26.
[4] Thorp JM, Richards WC, Telfer ABM. A survey of infection in an intensive care unit. *Anaesthesia* 1979;**34**:643–50.
[5] Campbell D. Immediate hospital care of the injured. *Br J Anaesth* 1977;**49**: 673–9.
[6] Trunkey DD. Inhalation injury. *Surg Clin North Am* 1978;**58**:1133–40.
[7] Edmondson RS, Flowers MW. Intensive care in tetanus: management, complications, and mortality in 100 cases, *Br Med J* 1979;i:1401–4.
[8] Golden FStC, Rivers JF. The immersion incident, *Anaesthesia* 1975;**30**: 364–73.
[9] Stoddart JC. Ventilatory management in the intensive therapy unit, *Br J Hosp Med* 1976;**16**:324–32.

Anaesthetists in the obstetric department

J SELWYN CRAWFORD

It is a characteristic of clinical practice within a hospital that the anaesthetist has the facility of being all things to all men, and that he (or almost as often, she) can restrict or extend his activities to suit the local demands and opportunities. The obstetric anaesthetist is no exception to this. In practical terms his role within a small obstetric unit will be very limited; in a larger unit his involvement will be deployed over a wider field, and its scope will become dependent on factors other than size, such as the quantitative and qualitative availability of anaesthetic and paediatric staff, and the degree of enthusiastic collaboration displayed by the obstetric and midwifery staff members.

There are five major areas of potential involvement: (*a*) the administration of anaesthesia for obstetric surgery; (*b*) consideration of systems for relieving pain in labour; (*c*) neonatal resuscitation; (*d*) intensive care of the seriously ill mother; and (*e*) intensive care of the seriously ill infant.

ANAESTHESIA FOR OBSTETRIC SURGERY

Initially, and for many decades, anaesthesia for obstetric surgery was almost the sole item of engagement by anaesthetists in obstetric units. With the exception of very few interested anaesthetists it was a tangential occupation, usually delegated to the on-call, under-trained junior anaesthetist (except for private patients), and accepted very much on sufferance by the anaesthetic establishment. Increasing appreciation of the challenges provided by obstetric patients and of the hazards to which anaesthesia exposes them, has helped to bring about a minor revolution.

The obstetric anaesthetist has now accepted the responsibility of not only providing anaesthesia (whether general or regional), but also of defining the prophylactic measures necessary to reduce the dangers associated with these activities and of rigorously supervising their sustained application. Such measures include the provision of appropriate diet, antacid prophylaxis, and advisable maternal posture during labour and delivery; the provision of anaesthetic help and advised apparatus at critical times such as induction of general anaesthesia; attention to fluid replacement and the anticipation of blood loss; and the provision of an appropriately equipped and staffed post-operative recovery room.

Anaesthetists in the obstetric department

RELIEF FROM PAIN IN LABOUR

Collaboration in the application and supervision of relief from pain and anxiety during labour has been an important part of obstetric anaesthetic practice. Although currently the provision of lumbar epidural analgesia has seized the public and professional imagination, the obstetric anaesthetist by no means confines his interest to that technique. He must have a mastery of all available means of providing relief from pain and anxiety—psychoprophylaxis and relaxation exercises, inhalational and systemically administered agents, and other techniques of local analgesia (including spinal and caudal block). In gaining this mastery he has to learn much that was not in his basic anaesthetic training. He learns that the pregnant woman differs considerably in many important respects from the "standard human subject." In her physiological characteristics, her metabolic responses (including her capacity to redistribute, metabolise, and excrete drugs), as well as in her anatomical features, she is truly a member of the "third sex."[1]

Additionally, the obstetric anaesthetist appreciates that the fetus is exposed to the effects of almost any treatment that he is likely to give the mother, and he must consequently have knowledge of placental physiology and the likely range of fetal responses. Protection against pain and anxiety in labour starts long before the mother enters the delivery suite. The obstetric anaesthetist co-operates with midwives, obstetric physiotherapists, and obstetricians in raising the confidence and self-assurance of the mother by contributing lectures and demonstrations in classes for antenatal preparation for childbirth. He also teaches pupil midwives—by obligatory formal lectures and informal demonstration and discourse—the elements of his and their common trade.

NEONATAL RESUSCITATION

Rough though reliable estimates suggest that, because of the deplorable lack of neonatologists in Britain, anaesthetists conduct about half of neonatal resuscitations. The anaesthetist, given his professional understanding of cardiorespiratory physiopathology and pharmacology, and his facility to intubate, is well equipped to fulfil this role. It may lead, however, to the potential danger of his having to look after two "at risk" patients simultaneously, and anaesthetists will welcome a considerable increase in a cadre of suitably experienced neonatologists to take over this responsibility.

Demarcation disputes have disappeared from all but a few antiquated centres, and there is general agreement that the depressed neonate should be resuscitated by the most experienced of the immediately available attendants (anaesthetist, paediatrician, or midwife). The anaesthetist is likely to maintain a role in teaching midwives and junior residents the elements of neonatal resuscitation.

INTENSIVE CARE OF THE SERIOUSLY ILL MOTHER

Intensive care of the seriously ill mother is well within the province of the obstetric anaesthetist, by virtue of his experience in non-obstetric intensive therapy units wedded to his understanding of the attributes of the "third sex." Most mothers in this category will be those with moderate or severe pre-eclampsia, but among the remainder will be those with a severe cardiac lesion, diabetes, renal disease, or disease of the central nervous system, as well as items of specific obstetric pathology. The greatest hazard to which such a mother can be exposed is that of consultation with a physician or surgeon who knows little about pregnancy.

In the absence of suitably experienced advice and help from non-obstetric colleagues, the obstetric anaesthetist should have the facility of adopting the role of general physician to the obstetric team. He will, in any event, collaborate with his obstetric and midwifery colleagues in constructing protocols to be followed during the care of seriously ill mothers and in furnishing—and maintaining in a state of preparedness—the full range of equipment and drugs that might be required for this purpose.

INTENSIVE CARE OF THE SERIOUSLY ILL INFANT

Somewhat similar remarks are applicable to the participation of the anaesthetist in the care of the critically ill infant, although here, historically, his interests have been limited mainly to the problems of ventilatory support. With the increasing and welcome tendency to regionalisation the anaesthetist's role here is diminishing, although he will doubtless continue to be a welcome adviser on matters of ventilator equipment and its application, and on the potential effects on the infant of drugs received and procedures undertaken before and during delivery.

OTHER RESPONSIBILITIES OF THE ANAESTHETIST

It will be seen that the potential role of the anaesthetist in an obstetric unit is a widely ranging one—as practising clinician, supervisor, teacher, and, above all, co-ordinator. He has other responsibilities as an administrator, not the least of which is that of supervising the maintenance of informative clinical records, so that successes and failures, and lessons learnt, will not be overlooked or forgotten. His work is probably the most important and professionally rewarding in the whole of anaesthetic practice, because half of his patients have potentially the longest life-span in the community, and the other half have the responsibility of rearing those in the first category to the age of their own responsibility. The onus is on our administrators and medical colleagues to make good the woeful insufficiency of committed obstetric anaesthetists in Britain.

REFERENCE

1 Crawford JS. *Principles and practice of obstetric anaesthesia.* 4th ed. Oxford: Blackwell, 1978:102.

The anaesthetist and the pain clinic

J W LLOYD

About 12 years ago there was an explosion in the topic of chronic pain management. Until that time, with the exception of opium which was first used in the third century BC, the field had been singularly barren. It is difficult to explain this long sterile period on the basis of pain being good for the soul, but indeed both Aristotle and Plato believed that pain was a passion of the soul and could be conquered by reason. The fact that this view was held for 2000 years did much to delay progress in the management of pain.

Pain remains today one of the most complex, irrational, and yet fascinating subjects in medicine. Technological advances and a greater understanding of the physiology and anatomy of pain have done much to further progress, but much is still empirical without scientific basis.

These gaps in our knowledge are being gradually filled in by experience gained largely in pain clinics that are now a feature of most large hospitals. Anaesthetists have taken the primary role in organising and managing these clinics, perhaps by virtue of their training, and in Britain run 98% of pain clinics.

Pain clinics are essentially outpatient clinics. If more than simple nerve blocks or the prescription of drugs is required lack of inpatient facilities becomes a limiting factor. Such facilities though desirable are by no means universally available. Clinics are broadly of three types: (1) pain clinic; (2) pain clinic with access to beds; and (3) a pain unit with autonomous control of beds.

Attendance at pain clinics is reserved for those suffering from intractable pain, and this may be defined as pain that has been present for over a month and is unremitting despite treatment. It is often associated with cancer, but this is misleading as many non-malignant conditions are equally capable of producing pain. In the Oxford Regional Pain Unit 28% of the patients admitted have pain of malignant origin. This contrasts with a figure of 70% ten years ago. Unfortunately it does not mean that cancer is on the decline but that the range of admissions has widened with a threefold increase in the total number of admissions (figure). This is perhaps indicative of the wider range of intractable pain now being tackled by pain clinics throughout the country. Referrals may be open or closed—that is, after specialist screening within the parent hospital. In the Oxford Regional Pain Unit the source of of referrals is general practitioner (40%), radiotherapist (25%), orthopaedic (15%), neurosurgical (12%), and miscellaneous (8%).

MANAGEMENT

Thorough assessment is of the utmost importance. It may be lengthy and require admission to hospital. This is often difficult in a general hospital and is best carried out in a pain relief unit which may have 8-10 beds for inpatients. The measurement of pain must still be subjective, but we find that observations over a few days of patients in the ward, coupled with their response to simple therapeutic tests, permit a useful degree of objectivity to be employed. This approach is of considerable value when dealing with patients who have a long history of a relatively trivial lesion, which over the years has been compounded by a large functional overlay. It may be argued that such patients can be effectively

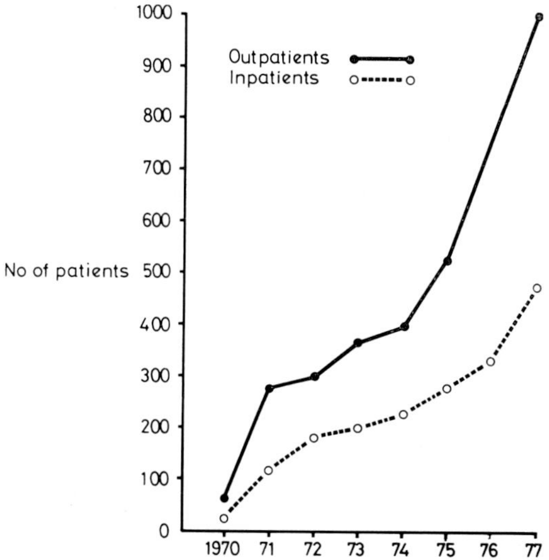

Numbers of inpatients and outpatients seen at pain relief unit 1970-7.

treated only in a unit that uses a multidisciplinary approach. Teaching is now an integral part of pain clinics. Research facilities, particularly for the collection of data, are becoming more available in the larger centres.

Unfortunately, pain relief units are not yet commonplace, though such a unit, attached to every teaching hospital authority, might add much to the management of these patients.

THE PROBLEM

Common presentations of intractable pain

Neuralgias—Trigeminal, intercostal, atypical facial, and myofascial syndrome.

Malignant disease—Carcinoma, myeloma, and lymphoma.

Reflex sympathetic dystrophies—Causalgia, phantom limb, and post-traumatic neuropathy.

Neurological disorders—Multiple sclerosis, spinal cord damage, syringomyelia, neurofibromatosis, neuromas, and nerve entrapment/damage.

Skeletal disorders—Osteoarthritis, lumbar disc syndrome, post-operative laminectomy pain, prolapsed disc, secondary neoplasm, and coccydynia.

Psychiatric disorders—A varying degree of functional disorder is found in 65% of patients attending the clinic. It is most common in the facial neuralgias and in those with chronic low back pain.

TREATMENT

The cornerstones of chronic pain relief are undoubtedly the use of drugs and the interruption of pain pathways by various means. It is important to realise that relief of intractable pain is not measured in terms of hours or days, but in months or years. It follows that the use of short-acting local anaesthetic drugs have diagnostic value alone.

Neurolytic agents

In Britain phenol and chlorocresol are commonly used quantitatively to destroy the nerves, and in successful cases this may relieve pain for 12–14 months. It is important to preserve motor function, and this is managed by using a concentration (5% phenol in glycerine) that selectively destroys the C fibres subserving pain and leaves the larger fibres intact.[1]

The solution is introduced into the subarachnoid space at the required dermatome level, and as it is hyperbaric from the addition of glycerine it falls as a result of gravity on to the required nerve roots. The patient can be tilted on the table to ensure accurate positioning. Some demyelination of the posterior columns may occur, but the increased activity consequent on pain relief more than compensates for the minimal weakness. The technique may be used at any level of the spinal cord but should be reserved, except in special conditions, for patients with malignant disease. Injections at the lower lumbar level carry a risk of bladder dysfunction that may not be acceptable to many patients.

Subarachnoid injections of alcohol are not popular in Britain, but the agent is of considerable value in destroying the sympathetic chain. Coeliac plexus block[2] with 50 ml of 50% alcohol is particularly effective in pain emanating from stomach, gall bladder, liver, and pancreas: 6% phenol in water is also used but more commonly to block the lumbar sympathetic chain in the reflex sympathetic dystrophies and in some cases of peripheral vascular insufficiency. The sympathetic dystrophy group should be regarded as emergencies as the chances of a successful result are inversely proportional to the time elapsing since they first occur. Injection of alcohol into the pituitary is a method introduced by Morrica,[3] and has successfully controlled pain from secondary bone deposits in hormone dependent tumour. One millilitre of dehydrated alcohol is introduced into the gland through a needle that is inserted through the nose and sphenoidal sinuses to the pituitary fossa. Pain is relieved so rapidly that it seems unlikely that a hormone mechanism can be postulated. There are now reports of success in relieving pain from non-hormone dependent tumours.

It is doubtful whether alcohol or phenol have any place in peripheral nerve blocks as the analgesia is commonly patchy, and there is a definite incidence of neuritis. One exception, however, is the injection of 40% alcohol into the muscle sheath of patients who have painful flexor spasms in multiple sclerosis.

Physical, electrical, and surgical methods of interrupting pain pathways

Physical, electrical, and surgical methods of interrupting pain pathways include replacement of the cerebrospinal fluid with ice cold saline,[4] barbotage of the cerebrospinal fluid,[5] percutaneous electrical cordotomy,[6] surgical sensory root rhizotomy,[7] surgical cordotomy,[8] cryoanalgesia,[9] transcutaneous nerve stimulation,[10] and acupuncture.

Replacement of the cerebrospinal fluid with ice cold saline and barbotage of the cerebrospinal fluid have a success rate of 45–50% with a duration of six to eight weeks. Both are remarkably free from complications, but replacing cerebrospinal fluid with ice cold saline is painful and needs an anaesthetic. Percutaneous electrical cordotomy is a valuable procedure producing excellent results in skilled hands. It is not generally practised in pain clinics but tends to be reserved for larger regional centres.

Cryoanalgesia is a new technique and provides a reversible block of transmission for 8–10 weeks. Interestingly, however, in cases of facial pain, comprising atypical facial neuralgia, post-traumatic neuropathies, postherpetic neuralgia, and trigeminal neuralgia, the duration of pain relief is considerably longer: 70% of these patients had pain relief for longer than six weeks and 50% for longer than six months. Three patients with tic douloureux had relief for more than three years. Clearly there is a central effect in operation as there was no evidence of a peripheral nerve block after 12 weeks. Both transcutaneous stimulation and acupuncture represent the move towards non-invasive methods of pain relief. Although attempts have been made to give scientific credence to the techniques, they have not gained universal acceptance. At the present state of our knowledge they must however be part of a pain clinic's armament.

The anaesthetist and the pain clinic

Drugs

All patients who attend pain clinics will have been taking analgesic drugs, many for a very long time indeed without any improvement in their symptoms.

Although not strictly analgesic, cytotoxic drugs, anti-inflammatory drugs, and steroids should be included in this group. The use of tranquillisers either alone or in conjunction with anticonvulsants or the phenothiazine group of drugs have also been useful in managing refractory pain problems.

Drugs are simple to administer, but effective prescribing demands considerable experience. The response to drugs is curiously personal, and it is well known that some patients with advanced cancer respond better to aspirin than to morphine. It would seem unrealistic to form a hard and fast drug regimen, and it may be more convenient to divide them into three groups (table).

Drugs for ambulant and non-ambulant patients

Ambulant patients

Group 1	Group 2
Acetyl salicylic acid (aspirin)	Dextromoramide (Palfium)
Dextropropoxyphene hydrochloride + paracetamol (Distalgesic)	Methadone (Physeptone)
Ethoheptazine + meprobomate (Equagesic)	Mefenamic acid (Ponstan)
Dihydrocodeine (DF118)	Levorphanol tartrate (Dromoran)
Paracetamol (Panadol) with DF118 (Paramol 118)	Pentazocine (Fortral)
Paracetamol + codeine (Paracodol)	Buprenorphine (Temgesic)
Diflunisal (Dolobid)	

Non-ambulant patients

Oxycodone pectinate (Proladone) suppositories
Dipipanone hydrochloride (Diconal)
Pethidine
Piritramide (Dipodolor)
Mist aspirin et nepenthe
Morphine
Diamorphine hydrochloride (heroin)
Brompton Hospital mixture (Hanstus E)

Tolerance to drugs, particularly the opiates, develops rapidly, and not uncommonly these patients need doses such as 120 mg of morphine every two hours after a comparatively short time. Doses of this magnitude, although necessary, are clearly undesirable, and it is in such cases that a nerve block, in combination with a drug, may allow reduction in the opiate and an improvement in the level of consciousness.

Drugs have the most important part to play in the later treatment of cancer pain when the disease becomes generalised. Because of the ease of administration they will, however, always be the first line of defence in treating pain.

In the final analysis it should be emphasised that although skill in performing nerve blocks and prescribing drugs is valuable, it is of minor importance compared with the proper understanding of the patient and his problems. The morale of these patients is balanced on a knife edge, and their care may be extremely difficult, demanding, and unrewarding. The correct management demands a multidisciplinary approach, inpatient facilities, and all the supportive treatment that this provides.

REFERENCES

1. Maher RM. Relief of pain in incurable cancer. *Lancet* 1955;i:18–20.
2. Bridenbaugh LD, Moore DC, Campbell DD. Management of upper abdominal cancer. *JAMA* 1964;**190**:877.
3. Moricca G. *Progress in anaesthesiology*. Amsterdam: Excerpta Medica, 1970:266–9.
4. Hitchcoock E. Hypothermic subarachnoid irrigation for intractable pain. *Lancet* 1967;i:1133–5.
5. Lloyd JW, Hughes JT, Davies-Jones GAB. Relief of severe intractable pain by barbotage of cerebrospinal fluid. *Lancet* 1972;i:354–5.
6. Lipton S. Percutaneous electrical cordotomy in relief of intractable pain. *Br Med J* 1968;ii:210–2.
7. White JC. Posterior rhizotomy: a possible substitute for cordotomy in otherwise intractable neuralgias of the trunk and extremities of non-malignant origin. *Clin Neurosurg* 1966;**13**:20–41.
8. Stookey B. The management of intractable pain by chordotomy. *Res Publ Ass Res Nerv Ment* 1943;**23**:416–33.
9. Lloyd JW, Barnard JDW, Glynn CJ. Cryoanalgesia, a new approach to pain relief. *Lancet* 1976;ii:932–4.
10. Wall PD, Sweet WH. Temporary abolition of pain in man. *Science* 1967;**155**:108–9.

The Committee on Review of Medicines

T B BINNS

In retrospect it is astonishing that until 1964 there was virtually no control over the marketing of drugs in Britain. In that year the voluntary Committee on Safety of Drugs (Dunlop Committee) came into operation, and when the Medicines Act of 1968 was finally implemented on September 1971 this was succeeded by the Committee on Safety of Medicines (CSM). The CSM advises the licensing authority, which is part of the medicines division of DHSS, on the granting of licences inter alia for clinical trials and new products. Products already on the market in September 1971 were given product licences of right. The data sheets on these products were prepared by the manufacturers, and very few of them had undergone independent evaluation.

Late in 1975 the Committee on Review of Medicines (CRM) was created to undertake this task and also to comply with an EEC directive that imposed a deadline for review of May 1990.[1] In status it corresponds to the CSM, being one of several committees set up under section 4 of the Medicines Act, and it operates in much the same way. Its members are appointed by the health ministers with the advice of the Medicines Commission. They are broadly representative of the interests concerned but are appointed as individuals and not as delegates. They are paid a nominal honorarium that is not remotely commensurate with the time taken up, so their decisions are in no way influenced by considerations of finance or job security. The first chairman was Sir Eric Scowen, and he was succeeded by Professor Owen Wade in 1979. Technically these committees report directly to the ministers, but there is a two-way traffic also with the Medicines Commission, the other section 4 committees, and the medicines division of DHSS, which provides the secretariat. Strictly speaking, it "advises" the licensing authority but the advice is usually acted on. Manufacturers may, however, appeal against decisions of the licensing authority based on this advice and may make representations either verbally or in writing. In the last resort they can request a hearing by the Medicines Commission.

At its inception the CRM faced a formidable task. Product licences of right had been issued for some 36 000 products, details of which were held on a computer. This figure is often bandied about as if all these were prescription products. In fact, it included about 10 000 herbal and 4000 homoeopathic products, many "home remedies," and some 12 000 so-called prescription fillers (generics sold under the name of the active ingredient without specific indications). There were more than 4000 proprietary medicines, but there could be as many as five or six licences for different dosage forms and strengths of the same drug. The most dramatic effect of the CRM was that by the end of 1976 some 10 000 licences were voluntarily surrendered, and many more products have since been withdrawn.

WORK OF THE CRM

Through the licensing authority the committee has very considerable powers affecting the composition, manufacture, supply, and labelling of products. It can restrict their use or even revoke licences.

It has had to decide various points of principle. For example, it did not pursue a proposal by the health ministers that it should categorise products into drugs at first, second, or reserve choice. It deferred consideration of homoeopathic products. It gave consideration to the use of drugs in children and set up a working group to advise on categories for their use in pregnancy. It formed subcommittees to deal systematically with particular therapeutic classes, giving priority where the need seemed greatest. The first three were on antirheumatic, analgesic, and psychotropic medicines. And it arranged that the biological subcommittee of the CSM should also serve the CRM.

The original systematic review procedure proved to be too protracted and was modified. In addition an accelerated review procedure was adopted whereby any drug or product could be considered as occasion demanded.

The remit of the committee is to consider and give advice with respect to the safety, quality, and efficacy in relation to human use of any substance or article to which any provision of the (Medicines) Act is applicable. It has to operate not only within these terms of reference but under various other constraints, such as shortage of professional staff, and with continual regard to external influences such as the EEC and WHO.

By law, therefore, all product licences should be reviewed according to these criteria, which are the same as those used by the CSM for evaluating new drugs. However, many of the preparations under review were originally introduced when testing and documentation were less advanced. It would be impractical to require them to be brought up to present-day standards and on the basis of past experience usually quite unnecessary apart from quality control data. There is a particular difficulty in applying the criteria to herbal and home remedies. It would be a pity to sweep away some of the comforting and harmless nostrums. Sometimes it is difficult to avoid adopting double standards, but each case is judged on its merits with a degree of common sense. Inevitably some inconsistencies and anomalies arise. At times it is necessary to consider a group of products together when some members of the group are borderline, but the committee is always ready to listen to manufacturers or trade associations and tries hard to be fair. The spirit of the old Dunlop Committee is still alive.

The committee is concerned with maintaining and improving standards, both in the quality of the products and in the information about them. This should be conducive to rational prescribing, but it is emphatically not concerned with restricting doctors' freedom to prescribe or otherwise control their use of drugs.

REFERENCE

[1] Penn RG. The review of medicines—a reappraisal of the older British drugs. *Health Trends* 1980;**12**:18–20.

The Committee on Safety of Medicines and the prescribing doctor

JAMES CROOKS

To understand the role of the Committee on Safety of Medicines and how its work contributes to that of the prescribing doctor it is helpful to ask what the doctor requires of a new medicine. The first requirement is that the drug should be efficacious in patients for whom the drug is indicated. The second requirement is that the drug should be safe, not in absolute terms since this is rarely possible but rather that the adverse effects produced by the drug should be identified as early as possible together with an estimate of the frequency of their occurrence so that the prescriber can apply a benefit/risk assessment as a component of the therapeutic decision to prescribe. The last requirement is that the quality of the medicine in respect of its formulation, manufacture and physical properties, route of administration, etc, should be of an acceptable standard.

When considering the role of the committee it should be appreciated that it is a statutory committee of independent experts which *gives advice* to the Licensing Authority (Health and Agricultural Ministers) concerning the acceptability of a new medicine to undergo clinical trials or be granted a product licence that would allow it to be marketed. A pharmaceutical company may appeal, under the Medicines Act of 1968, to the Medicines Commission against this advice.

Thus I have emphasised the advisory function of the committee, but how does it ensure that the prescribing doctor will have available new medicines that are efficacious, safe, and of acceptable quality? It does this in the following way. First of all it subjects a new drug to an assessment procedure before *recommending* that it is given a clinical trial certificate. It then takes into account all the information made available by the sponsoring company including the clinical trial results before *recommending* that it be given a product licence, which allows it to be marketed. Lastly, the committee maintains its interest in ensuring that prescribers have safe and effective drugs at their disposal by organising postmarketing surveillance of new drugs in terms of adverse reactions, product manufacturing defects, advertising controls, and the provision of information to prescribing doctors about drug problems as they arise. The committee does much of this work helped by several expert subcommittees.

CLINICAL TRIAL CERTIFICATE

Before clinical trials may be performed with a new drug never before available or for a new indication for a drug already on the market a company must submit details of the drug to the Committee on Safety of Medicines. To grant a clinical trial certificate the committee must be satisfied that studies of the drug in animals and in human volunteers show adequate promise of therapeutic potential. Special attention is paid to the toxicity of the drug in both the animal and human studies. The former provides data on potential mutagenicity and carcinogenicity that are of particular importance when the chemical group to which the drug belongs, the indications for its use, and the type of drug regimen proposed suggest that there may be a problem. The pharmaceutical aspects of the formulation are also assessed to conform with agreed standards of purity in respect of the drug and other substances in the formulation.

The clinicians and centres carrying out the clinical trial have also to be acceptable to the committee, which has to try to achieve flexibility in its criteria for acceptable clinical trials to avoid inhibiting new drug development. It also has to try to ensure that the results of the trial will provide the scientific evidence that will allow it to reach a satisfactory decision on the allocation of a product licence.

PRODUCT LICENCE

In granting a product licence the committee must be satisfied that the doctor can prescribe a drug secure in the knowledge that so far as is reasonably possible the drug has been shown to be both safe and effective as judged by animal studies and clinical trials and that all available evidence suggests that this will be maintained when the drug becomes generally available. It would be reasonable to say that the decision about the efficacy of the drug is usually resolved by the results of the clinical trials, provided the protocol has been satisfactory and the trial well executed.

The question of safety presents greater problems, and the committee goes to great lengths in making decisions over safety, particularly in respect of the extrapolation of toxicological studies in animals to man. Their concern over the problem was manifest by its sponsorship of an international conference on the validity of extrapolating to man the carcinogenic properties of drugs to produce breast cancer in beagle dogs. After consideration of a large amount of evidence the conclusion was reached that the extrapolation was not valid. The amount of effort expended by the committee on problems such as this must be reassuring to both the prescribing doctor and the patient.

POSTMARKETING SURVEILLANCE

It has been appreciated in recent years that the price to be paid by the community for having effective drugs made available is that a few of these drugs may produce serious adverse effects, which, though rare, would require removal of the drug from the market—for instance, thalidomide and practolol. It is also clear that toxicological data derived from animal studies may not provide information to predict this and because of the rarity of the reactions conventional clinical trials cannot be expected to do so. It follows that the postmarketing period of drug development should be monitored to detect clinically important adverse effects. Through its adverse reactions subcommittee the committee attempts to do this by its "yellow card" system, in which the doctor is requested to report any suspected adverse reaction that is new or serious. The co-operation of prescribing doctors with the committee has resulted in the British system of voluntary reporting of adverse reactions being the most effective in the world. This view must be tempered by the fact that under 1% of serious previously unsuspected adverse effects are reported under this system—for instance, thromboembolism and the oral contraceptives—and to improve this voluntary reporting system prescribing doctors must recognise their responsibility to report suspected adverse effects on the yellow cards if both they and the committee are to attain their mutual objective of increased safety of drugs for patients. It should be emphasised that, although summaries of the register of adverse reactions or excerpts from it are available to bona-fide inquiries, the name of the patient and the doctor concerned are always kept confidential. As well as the yellow card system the committee monitors adverse reaction reports from a variety of sources including the pharmaceutical industry, other countries through the World Health Organisation, and medical publications.

The committee can also *recommend* that a particular medicine should be given a product licence that will allow it to be marketed but on condition that the sponsoring company sets up a "monitored release" procedure. This means that the company must take special steps, using a method and time scale agreed by the committee, to monitor the use of the medicine in terms, for example, of adverse reactions and the appropriateness of the indications for use. Postmarketing surveillance of a new drug also includes continuing scrutiny of the manufacturing procedure by the licensing authority to ensure the maintenance of pharmaceutical quality.

The committee has also been considering the feasibility of developing new methods for postmarketing surveillance of drugs using, for example, the data provided by the prescription-pricing authority, but the choice of the most appropriate system is difficult because of the need to justify "cost effectiveness." Nevertheless, further developments can be expected on this aspect.

COMMUNICATION BETWEEN THE COMMITTEE AND THE PRESCRIBING DOCTOR

An important part of the committee's work is directed towards providing the prescribing doctor with information that will allow him to identify problems that have been derived from "yellow card" reporting or other information sources. The methods of doing this depend on the type of problem and the urgency of finding a solution. For example, leaflets in the "Adverse Reactions Series" are issued to all doctors and dentists when it is necessary to give urgent warnings about an adverse reaction. For less urgent problems the committee chairman usually sends "Dear Doctor" letters, outlining the nature of the problem. When potential future problems in drug treatment are identified by the committee but where there is an absence of conclusive evidence that would allow appropriate advice to be given to prescribers the mechanism of communication used is the issue to doctors of a leaflet headed "Current Problems." The intention of this communication is to inform him of the nature of the problem (perhaps an adverse effect suspected but not conclusively) associated with the administration of a particular drug. It is hoped that the doctors' threshold for the detection of a possible association will change, although it should be emphasised that the interpretation of an increased number of reports after such a communication takes account of the changed circumstances.

The committee not infrequently uses other methods of informing doctors about drug problems—for instance, through the medical press and the manufacturers' publications. In the case of the latter the committee keeps under review the postmarketing performance of new licensed drugs, and if in their view the data sheet, which provides the information the pharmaceutical company must provide to doctors, requires amendment they *recommend* that this should be done. The committee also *advises* the Licensing Authority when, in their view, the promotion of the product, through advertising material, is not compatible with the claims made for the medicine in the data sheet that the committee have accepted as reasonable. The way in which the committee operates and its responsibilities to government, the medical profession, and the public needs to be understood by all three but especially by the prescribing doctor.

Drug development

CHARLES F GEORGE

Currently between 15 and 20 new medicines (as opposed to new formulations of old drugs) are marketed in an average year. Before the introduction of any drug to man, many months and usually several years of research and development have taken place. The starting point for discovery of a new drug may be reached in several different ways. Firstly, chemical entities that have been synthesised by the same or another company are subjected to a battery of tests designed to detect different types of biological activity. These include studies of the effects on animal behaviour and work on isolated tissues. In addition animal models of disease states are sometimes used. In general this is not an efficient form of research since at best only one in every four to five thousand chemical entities screened is marketed as a medicine. Indeed, recent evidence suggests the ratio may be closer to one in ten thousand: it is for this reason that this "random" approach is losing favour.

A second approach entails the synthesis and testing of chemical analogues of existing medicines for biological activity. Although in general this leads to minor advantages such as better absorption, greater potency, and a more selective action, surprises may occur. On occasions these are disadvantageous and may limit the subsequent use of the drug. Additional properties, however, may become evident when the compound is tried in man. This serendipitous approach led to the introduction of the thiazide diuretics and oral hypoglycaemic agents (both of which represent slight modifications of the early antimicrobial sulphanilamide) and of clonidine for hypertension.

The newest and most rational form of research and development has been to design a substance to fulfil a particular biological role. At its simplest this may entail the synthesis of a naturally occurring substance —for example, a hormone or vitamin. A good example is the introduction of levodopa, a precursor of the neurotransmitter dopamine, which is deficient in patients with Parkinson's disease.

Alternatively, chemical analogues of naturally occurring substances have been developed with the intent of modifying the effects of the endogenous substances. Drugs of this type include the beta-adrenoceptor antagonists (initially pronethalol and propranolol) to block the effects of circulating catecholamines and thereby reduce myocardial oxygen consumption to relieve angina pectoris. More recent examples include cimetidine to block the action of histamine on H_2 receptors, thus reducing acid output from the stomach to allow healing of peptic ulcers. Captopril is another substance introduced recently to inhibit the action of the converting enzyme responsible for generating angiotensin II, thereby lowering blood pressure.

Although this approach has been successful in recent years, the main problem limiting the rate of introduction of new drugs on a "logical" basis is the lack of understanding of basic physiological and biochemical processes (as well as the homeostatic mechanisms that will be brought into play when the "milieu intérieur" is disturbed).

A fourth approach, in which there is renewed interest, is the re-investigation of traditional, usually herbal, remedies for their active ingredients. Although most remedies that have been in use for generations are pharmacologically useless, from them a few chemicals have been identified that may become useful either in synthetic or in semisynthetic form.

PRECLINICAL TESTING

Before a "new product candidate" can be tried in man several months or years must be spent on toxicological studies, the development of analytical techniques, and metabolic studies. These are necessary to allow the prediction of what will be the effective dose in man and to minimise the risks. Countries differ in their requirements for toxicity testing, but in general the following procedures will be necessary.

There are three main phases: firstly, acute studies in which the dose required to kill half of a group of animals from two or three species after a single administration is established: gross pathological changes are then noted. Secondly, subacute studies require the regular administration of the drug (by the same route as it is intended to use the product in man) in two or three animal species for up to 90 days. Organ function is measured, and not only is the gross pathology studied but also microscopic anatomy. Thirdly, chronic studies necessitate administering the drug to two or three animal species for at least six months. Similar measurements are made to those listed for subacute toxicity, but in addition studies of reproductive capacity and mutagenicity are usually required.

Examples in which animal toxicity data have been of good predictive value for man are the peripheral neuropathy associated with the use of isoniazid and both renal toxicity and ototoxicity associated with the aminoglycoside antibiotics. False predictions, however, may occur because of rapid excretion in animals, differences in their pathways of metabolism, receptor sensitivity, anatomy and physiology, and as a result of the lack of pre-existing pathology. Although toxicological testing is performed routinely, it has no absolute predictive value for adverse reactions in man. Examples of toxicity not seen in animals include the oculomucocutaneous syndrome seen with regular ingestion of practolol and the cutaneous and renal problems associated with the use of captopril. The only way to find out whether a new drug is safe in man is to give it to him: some risk is unavoidable if new drugs are to become available for treating diseases that either do not respond at all or for which existing treatment is unsatisfactory.

CLINICAL STUDIES

The purposes of clinical studies are, firstly, to establish that a drug has a useful action in man; secondly, to confirm that it is non-toxic; and, thirdly, to establish the nature of common side effects. It is conventional to subdivide the clinical testing into three phases, but the distinction between these is blurred and not everyone agrees on the classification that I shall use.

Phase I studies

Phase I studies is a term used to describe the first few administrations of a new drug to man. The precise conduct of these studies varies according to the type of drug being studied and whether the investigator is based in academic medicine or the pharmaceutical industry. The choice of subjects for phase I studies is normally "volunteers" recruited from within the pharmaceutical industry or by open advertisement.

The first few administrations are usually swallowed in a dose of 1/50th of the minimum required to produce some effect in animals.[1] In future, however, increasing use will probably be made of intravenous administration, since the disposition and fate of the drug as well as its actions may be studied more easily. Depending on findings obtained in animals, the dose may then be built up in man either by using small increments or doubling until either a pharmacological effect is seen or an unwanted effect occurs. One of the main objects of phase I studies is to screen for possible toxic effects; it is therefore usual to make routine haematological measurements and biochemical estimations of liver and renal function, as well as to perform routine urine analysis. Additional tests might be indicated if an analogue of the drug under study had produced a particular form of toxicity—for example, looking for DNA antibodies.

It is usual practice to study the disposition, metabolism, and main pathways of elimination of drugs at this early stage of development.[2] Not only does this add precision to the choice of dose for subsequent study but also it may help to identify which animal species handles the drug in a manner similar to man. (This species might then be used during long-term toxicity studies.) Investigations on drug metabolism and pharmacokinetics often necessitate the use of beta-emitting compounds such as ^{14}C or ^{3}H or alternatively stable isotopes such as deuterium.

Phase 2 studies

In phase 2 the clinical pharmacology of the new drug is studied by a few designated investigators chosen for their training and skill. These doctors will have taken part in drawing up the protocol and should have submitted this to the local ethics committee. The design of the protocol to be followed will depend on the type of drug under study. In assessing a new antihypertensive, for example, patients might be given a placebo on the first day of study and recordings made of the pulse and blood pressure at 30-minute intervals both supine and erect for eight hours or so thereafter. Increasing doses of the new drug would then be given on succeeding days to establish whether it had an acute hypotensive effect and to gain some idea of the slope of its dose-response curve. Additional pharmacological studies could be undertaken to show that the hypotensive action was that predicted from animal studies—for example, methyldopa was introduced because of its ability to block dopa decarboxylase in animals, but it lowers blood pressure by a different action in man. If the blood pressure had been satisfactorily reduced during the initial studies the patient could then be started on a maintenance dose of the drug and any further adjustments made at regular outpatient attendances.

Often the initial assessment of drugs in phase 2 is done on an open basis. Although the results of such studies may suggest that a new drug has efficacy, this form of evaluation does not prove that it works. Some existing remedies (as well as many more that have since been discarded) were subjected to this empirical type of approach and the fact that diseases are dynamic (undergoing continuous change in their natural history) was not taken into account. Furthermore, the large subjective element in many illnesses means that more than one-third of patients respond favourably to any intervention. To prove that a drug has efficacy it is necessary to undertake formal clinical trials.

Phase 3 studies

Formal clinical trials seek, firstly, to establish whether a new drug works in comparison with a placebo that looks (and tastes) identical with the active compound. Secondly, they aim at establishing the advantages and disadvantages by comparison with the best available treatment. For example, with a new antihypertensive drug it would be appropriate to compare it with either methyldopa or a diuretic. Similarly, a new anti-inflammatory analgesic might be compared with aspirin or indomethacin. It is beyond the remit of this article to discuss clinical trials in detail. Suffice it to say that there are two main types: within patient "cross-over" studies or between patient comparisons.[3] The latter may be performed on either a fixed number, chosen according to likely predictions,[4] or using a sequential design.

The results of treatment with a new product are assessed by a combination of objective and subjective techniques. Pulse, blood pressure, size of finger joint, strength of grip, and the number of additional analgesic tablets, such as paracetamol, required to control pain represent objective measurements. Subjective measurements would include the duration of morning stiffness and the intensity of pain. Visual analogue rating scales have become a popular (and surprisingly accurate) way of assessing many subjective effects, such as pain relief, and may be used also to assess side effects, such as sedation.

Marketing of the new drug

Once sufficient clinical and preclinical data have been collected on the safety and efficacy of a new chemical, submission is made to the Committee on Safety of Medicines. If the information provided is satisfactory a product licence can then be issued. By this time ten or more years may have elapsed since the taking out of a patent on the "new product candidate" and a total of £20m expended. Only a few hundred patients, however, will have been exposed to the drug. Thus the full benefits and problems associated with its use may not become apparent until months or years after it has been marketed. Because of the latter possibility I would suggest that practitioners should adopt a cautious attitude towards new medicines. In my view there is no justification for switching automatically to the 15th "β-blocker" from one that has been in use for ten years or more, since it is unlikely that the new compound will have a measurable advantage for most patients. Possibly, however, it may have advantages for some patients—for example, a cardioselective β-adrenoceptor antagonist would be preferable to propranolol if the patient had coexistent airways obstruction or diabetes mellitus. Similarly, a tetracyclic antidepressant might be preferable for a patient with coexistent cardiac disease.

In addition my personal rule is to insist that there are at least two good clinical studies (with similar results) showing that the drug has therapeutic (rather than just statistically significant) advantages in a particular condition before prescribing it.

REFERENCES

1 Dollery CT, Davies DS. Conduct of initial drug studies in man. *Br Med Bull* 1970;**26**:233–6.

2 Downie CC. Clinical pharmacology. In: Harris EL, Fitzgerald JD, eds. *The principles and practice of clinical trials*. Edinburgh and London: Livingstone, 1970;15–22.

3 George CF. The investigation of new drugs in man. *Br J Hosp Med* 1974;**12**: 780–9.

4 Clark CJ, Downie CC. A method for the rapid determination of the number of patients to include in a controlled clinical trial. *Lancet* 1966;ii:1357–8.

Drug monitoring

D C MOIR

The practice of medicine has been transformed in recent years by the marketing of many pharmacologically active and therapeutically effective drugs. Unfortunately, however, the administration of some of these compounds has produced unwanted effects, and concern about the best ways of recognising these has repeatedly been expressed. This concern has increased more in recent years with the recognition of an association between practolol and an oculomucocutaneous syndrome,[1] and attention has been drawn to the deficiencies in the existing systems for detecting these unwanted adverse effects.

Increasingly stringent toxicological investigation of all new drugs is carried out in animals and, if satisfactory, is followed by clinical trials. Nevertheless, such methods detect only the more common and predictable side effects and are inadequate for identifying the infrequent and unpredictable adverse drug reactions that become apparent only after several years of unrestricted clinical use.

The primary objective in drug monitoring is to diminish the period between the general release of a drug and the full recognition of its ability to produce undesirable side effects. This objective can be met only if two facilities are available: firstly, a means of recognising previously unsuspected adverse reactions and, secondly, a procedure whereby the suspicion can be confirmed or refuted and if confirmed the frequency and severity of the adverse effect determined.

METHODS OF DETECTION

Two main methods of detecting adverse reactions have been developed—voluntary reporting systems and intensive surveillance of defined hospital populations.

Voluntary reporting

Voluntary reporting systems, such as the "yellow card"[2] early warning system operated by the Committee on Safety of Medicines in Britain, have met with limited success. The low yield from doctors in particular seems illogical, since so many new drugs are prescribed initially in hospital and many of the major reactions occurring outside hospital necessitate admission to hospital. Despite the low level of reporting, clustering of reports around a drug can provide early warning of an unsuspected effect. The subcommittee on adverse reactions of the Committee on Safety of Medicines also examines the patterns of adverse drug reactions produced by chemically similar drugs. While these profiles are often similar for related drugs, on occasion one drug may present with a relatively much larger proportion of a specific adverse reaction and in this way previously unsuspected reactions can be signalled.

Since the likelihood of complete spontaneous reporting is remote and the number of people using the drug and who are, therefore, at risk, is unknown, the system can be of limited value only and cannot provide evidence of a causal relationship between a drug and a side effect. Similar systems, however, operate in several other countries, and 23 of these submit data in the same format to the World Health Organisation International Project on Drug Monitoring.[3] The value of this technique is enhanced by such international collaboration; the data is computerised and subjected to complex statistical programs that facilitate the signalling of unsuspected reactions earlier than would have been possible in the individual countries. While there are undoubtedly problems in interpreting such data, inferences may be drawn provided there is an awareness of the constraints that surround the collection and validation of such data in the individual countries. At the present time voluntary reporting systems still have a part to play in detecting previously unsuspected reactions.

Intensive surveillance

Intensive surveillance concentrates on the reporting by a designated group of doctors, nurses, or pharmacists screening a defined population for the specific purpose of ascertaining adverse drug reactions. Adverse reactions can be identified in this way since both the number of adverse events and the number receiving the drug are known, and this has been demonstrated by the Boston Collaborative Drug Surveillance Program.[4] Adverse effects, however, are fortunately relatively rare and because of the limited period in hospital there are practical difficulties in identifying adverse reactions which may not occur in the relatively small population that can be studied in this way, or which may not become apparent for some considerable time after the initial administration of the drug. Indeed, the cost and organisational complexity of this approach limits its wider application in the routine detection of adverse drug reactions.

In Britain the Medicines Evaluation and Monitoring Group (MEMO)[5] have devised a simple and relatively cheap method of identifying the total population who have received a drug or combination of drugs prescribed in hospital. The drugs prescribed are linked with patient vital statistic data and held on a computer file, and, since the file contains data on some 50 000 patients discharged annually from acute general hospitals, it is possible to investigate the occurrence of a suspected effect in a population receiving the suspect drug and in a suitably matched control population who did not receive the drug in question. Thus suspicions raised by voluntary reporting schemes or intensive surveillance may be rapidly confirmed or refuted.

POSSIBLE IMPROVEMENTS

Recorded release

While these systems go some way towards meeting the objectives of drug monitoring, various proposals have recently been made as to how the existing arrangements could be improved, and all of them necessitate ascertainment of cohorts of patients. Inman has advocated recorded release,[6] whereby new drugs would be given a provisional licence for use in recorded patients. Any doctor would be free to prescribe them provided he was prepared to provide the Committee on Safety of Medicines with a copy of the prescription plus basic clinical information. Subsequently the doctor would be asked to complete a second form recording any unexpected events that had occurred during treatment.

Rawlins and Dollery[7] proposed a similar scheme, registered release, excepting that the patient should be asked to complete the questionnaire, while Lawson[8] suggested a scheme in which the dispensing pharmacist would record the names of patients receiving new drugs. Similar arrangements are operating in selected hospitals in England, where hospital pharmacists report untoward events on several selected drugs. One weakness of such systems is the lack of suitable controls to compare with those patients receiving the new drugs while the numbers studied in such schemes tend to be too small and the period over which they run too short to identify adverse reactions that occur infrequently.

Prescription perusal

Another method of obtaining cohorts of patients receiving specified drugs is through the Prescription Pricing Authority in England[9] and the Pricing Bureau in Scotland. Prescriptions, written by general practitioners on FP10 and EC10 in England and Scotland, respectively, are dispensed by retail pharmacists and forwarded routinely to DHSS and the Scottish Home and Health Department as part of the scheme for reimbursing pharmacists. The identification of patients receiving specified drugs by way of a system in operation for another purpose has obvious attractions, and studies are in progress to determine the feasibility of using this method to identify patients for investigating suspected adverse reactions. As most drugs are taken in the community initial experiments with a repeat prescribing system suggest that they may prove to be a practical method of identifying patients taking long-term drugs. If these methods of identifying groups at risk prove satisfactory, consideration will then have to be given to the frequency with which the groups are followed up and the duration of routine follow-up. These will influence the cost of using this method as a monitoring tool; such types of monitoring must not, however, be restricted solely to new drugs, for drugs on the market for many years may prove to have long-delayed effects.

Record linkage

The feasibility of using record linkage, whereby records of major events such as births, deaths, admissions to hospital, and obstetric deliveries are linked for a population in a particular area has also been investigated using the Oxford Record Linkage Study[10] set up by Acheson in 1962. In 1974 basic information from this study including records of morbidity and mortality was linked with details provided by the Prescription Pricing Authority of the drugs dispensed, and the data were thereafter analysed for statistically significant associations between drugs and events, as has been shown by Skegg and Doll[11] for practolol and the frequency of eye complaints. This system is particularly relevant to identifying delayed effects, but it must be remembered that it does not include drugs given in hospital.

OPCS records

The records of births and deaths collected by the Office of Population, Censuses and Surveys (OPCS)[12] may also be used to study changes in the patterns of causes of deaths, and in this way suspicions linking a particular disease with a possible treatment may be raised. While there are undoubtedly problems as to the accuracy of such records and the information cannot be used in isolation, nevertheless, taken in conjunction with what is already known about a drug or chemically related compound, it may be used to provide further insights into the occurrence of possible adverse effects. In particular the linkage of OPCS data with National Health Service Register Numbers in the National Cancer Registry has potential for identifying delayed carcinogenic effects. The OPCS already maintains a register of congenital malformations, and this may be used to investigate malformations that are suspected of having an association with a drug administered during pregnancy. The possible association of congenital malformations with the administration of Debendox[13] has recently been investigated in Northern Ireland using the Registrar General's data on births and congenital malformations over several years and correlating it with the number of prescriptions written for Debendox. While the number of prescriptions rose, the incidence of congenital deformities decreased, suggesting that there is no evidence to support the suspected association.

CRITERIA OF SUCCESS

All of these systems have the ability to generate hypotheses that the administration of a drug may be linked with the occurrence of a particular unexplained event. Their success, as measured by the speed with which the adverse effect is detected after marketing, will also be determined by the frequency and severity with which the adverse effect occurs. For if the reaction is very infrequent, albeit serious, large populations will need to be studied before there is any hope of identifying low-frequency reactions. The problems may be further compounded by multiple drug prescribing, and factors such as age, sex, and genetic constitution may play a part in an individual's susceptibility to develop an adverse reaction.

Such systems can never establish with certainty the cause and effect relationship between a drug and unexplained event: this requires the detailed pharmacological investigation that is the necessary complement to drug monitoring. While epidemiological techniques could probably play a part in determining the safer use of drugs, questions have recently been raised in the House of Commons regarding the cost effectiveness and hence practicability of retrospective assessment of drug safety (RADS) and record linkage in the present economic climate.

The ultimate success of any scheme depends on an effective method of communicating relevant information to members of the health professions and in some instances to patients. It is essential that those concerned in investigating suspected hazards must not be pressurised to publish their findings prematurely while, on the other hand, they have a responsibility to act if a serious hazard occurs. The seriousness of any drug hazard will finally be judged in relation to the disease for which the drug is prescribed. While minor adverse effects may not be tolerable for drugs used to treat minor symptoms, more serious reactions may be tolerated if the disease for which they are prescribed is life threatening.

REFERENCES

1 Wright P. Untoward effects associated with practolol administration: oculomucocutaneous syndrome. *Br Med J* 1975;i:595–8.

2 Inman WHW. Monitoring by voluntary reporting at national level. In: Richards DJ, Rondel RK, eds. *Adverse drug reactions*. London: Churchill Livingstone, 1972:86–102.

3 Royall BW. International aspects of drug monitoring: role of the World Health Organisation. *WHO Chron* 1971;**25**:445–51.

4 Slone D, Jick H, Borda I, *et al*. Drug surveillance utilising nurse monitors: an epidemiological approach. *Lancet* 1966;ii:901–3.

5 Moir DC, Alexander ER, Barnett JW, Christopher LJ. A hospital based drug information system. *Health Bull* (*Edinb*) 1975;**33**:82–8.

6 Inman WHW. *Recorded release*. In: Gross FH, Inman WHW, eds. *Drug monitoring*. London: Academic Press, 1977:65–75.

7 Rawlins MD, Dollery CT. Post-marketing surveillance by registered release. In: *Post-marketing surveillance of adverse reactions to new medicines*. London: Medico-pharmaceutical Forum, 1978:40–4. (Publication No 7.)

8 Lawson DH. Post-marketing surveillance: an alternative approach. In: *Post-marketing surveillance of adverse reactions to new medicines*. London: Medico-pharmaceutical Forum, 1978:50–5. (Publication No 7.)

[9] Anonymous. Life cycle of an FP10. *Br Med J* 1977;ii:670.
[10] Acheson ED. *Medical record linkage.* London: Oxford University Press, 1967.
[11] Skegg DCG, Doll R. Frequency of eye complaints and rashes among patients receiving practotol and propranolol. *Lancet* 1977;ii:475–8.
[12] Dollery CT, Rawlins MD. Monitoring adverse reactions to drugs. *Br Med J* 1977;i:96–7.
[13] Harron DWG, Griffiths K, Shanks RG. Debendox and congenital malformations in Northern Ireland. *Br Med J* 1980;**281**:1379–81.

Drug absorption

A K SCOTT, GABRIELLE M HAWKSWORTH

The bioavailability of ingested drugs is influenced both by absorption and by the extent of metabolism occurring in the first pass through the liver As most drugs are swallowed, the emphasis in this article will be on absorption from the gastrointestinal tract with a brief reference to the problems associated with intramuscular injection.

Drug absorption is governed mainly by the physicochemical properties of the drug—in particular its lipid solubility, the degree of ionisation, and its molecular size. Lipid soluble drugs are well absorbed across the mucosal cells by passive diffusion. The absorption of drugs that are weak acids or weak bases is, in addition, determined by their dissociation constant and the pH of the environment. Acidic drugs will be mostly unionised in an acid medium and, since cell membranes are freely permeable only to the unionised form of a drug, acidic drugs, such as aspirin, phenobarbitone, and warfarin, should be better absorbed from the gastric contents than from the more neutral upper small intestine. The converse would apply for basic drugs—for instance, propranolol or imipramine. In practice, many weakly acidic drugs are better absorbed from the upper small intestine than from the stomach, owing to the greater absorptive surface of the small intestine and also partly because drugs such as aspirin are more soluble in neutral or alkaline solutions than in acidic solutions. Drugs that are strong acids or bases—for instance, quarternary ammonium compounds such as neostigmine—are completely ionised in aqueous solution and therefore poorly absorbed from all regions of the gut.

Some drugs are designed for minimal absorption in order to exert their pharmacological effect in the large intestine—for instance, the prodrug sulphasalazine—which is metabolised by the intestinal bacteria in the colon to liberate sulphapyridine and 5-aminosalicylate. Although most drugs are absorbed by passive diffusion, vitamins and drugs related to the steroids, amino-acids, or pyrimidines—for instance, levodopa—may be absorbed by active processes normally involved in the absorption of endogenous substances.

FORMULATION

For solid dosage formulations two other factors must be taken into consideration—*drug disintegration* and *drug dissolution*. Only drugs that are in solution will be absorbed, and the dissolution rate may vary greatly depending on the formulation or the drug salt used. After the problems with altered response and toxicity due to different formulations of phenytoin and digoxin much has been said of the need to use a particular brand of various drugs. Pharmacokinetic studies have shown differences in bioavailability among various brands of a wide range of drugs. In practice, the changes noted are of little or no clinical significance for most drugs. Formulation requires more serious consideration when using drugs with a narrow therapeutic index, such as phenytoin, digoxin, lithium, and warfarin, where a small change in bioavailability may alter the drug concentration to a level outside its therapeutically useful range. When using these drugs the same formulation should be adhered to throughout treatment.

Some drugs, notably penicillin G and erythromycin, are unstable in an acid environment and therefore their bioavailability is low after oral administration. Penicillins with a modified side chain attached to 6-aminopenicillanic acid, such as ampicillin, are better absorbed from the gastrointestinal tract, but in addition have a different antibacterial spectrum. Enteric-coated formulations of erythromycin are available, which protect the drug from the acidic stomach secretions. In other cases enteric coating may be used to protect the stomach from the irritant effect of the drug, as with aspirin or iron preparations. Sustained-release formulations are also available, but these are useful only for drugs with a large therapeutic index, a biological half life of three to eight hours, and for those drugs that are not absorbed by active processes. Drugs such as propranolol and theophylline have proved to be suitable candidates for sustained-release formulation.

GASTRIC MOTILITY

A decrease in gastric motility will tend to slow the *rate*, but not alter the *extent* of drug absorption. Differences in absorption rate are important when an immediate effect is required, as with analgesics or hypnotics, but are unimportant for drugs administered chronically, as *steady-state* drug concentrations do not change. Anticholinergics and antihistamines delay gastric emptying due to their atropine-like effects and may decrease the rate of absorption of a concomitantly administered drug. Examples of drugs causing an increase in the rate of gastric emptying are few—for instance, metoclopramide (see drug-drug interactions below).

FOOD AND FLUID VOLUME

Many of the effects of food on drug bioavailability may be explained in terms of effects on gastric emptying. The presence of food in the stomach delays gastric emptying, and this may slow down drug absorption. The total absorption of several antibiotics—for instance, penicillins, erythromycin, and tetracyclines—is decreased when given with food, and these drugs should be administered at least one hour before or three hours after meals. In the case of acid-labile penicillins and erythromycin the decreased absorption is partly due to prolonged time in the stomach, which results in increased degradation of the drug. Tetracyclines may undergo chelation with metal ions present in the diet, and this will impair absorption.

Fluid volume appears to have a considerable effect on drug absorption, most drugs being better absorbed when taken with an increased volume of water. This may be due to more rapid stomach emptying of large volumes of fluid, or, for drugs in solid dosage forms, to increased dissolution of drugs that are not freely water soluble.

DISEASE

The effect of gastrointestinal and systemic disease on drug absorption has not been extensively studied. As mentioned, diseases altering gastric motility will not affect the extent of drug absorption. The gastrointestinal tract has a large surface area, and for most drugs problems with absorption would be expected only in severe malabsorption disorders, as in some cases of coeliac disease or extensive small bowel resection. Absorption may be more seriously altered for drugs that are absorbed primarily from a localised area of the small intestine—for instance, iron from the duodenum and upper jejunum (reduced in enteropathy) and B_{12} from the terminal ileum (reduced in Crohn's disease). It has been suggested that oral contraceptives might fail if an episode of diarrhoea decreases the enterohepatic circulation of the oestrogen component. Liver disease with biliary obstruction may reduce the absorption of some fat-soluble drugs, but for most drugs the effects on first-pass metabolism and drug clearance are more important than a change in absorption.

Congestive cardiac failure delays absorption of some drugs—for instance, thiazide diuretics, quinidine, and digoxin—possibly owing to oedema of the intestinal mucosa or to decreased splanchnic blood flow. In practice, it is not usually necessary to alter drug dosage because of theoretical considerations of impaired drug absorption in disease states.

AGE

Until recent years there has been little interest in the absorption of drugs in the elderly. Studies suggest that for drugs that are absorbed by passive diffusion there is no appreciable change with age. Drugs absorbed by an active process, such as methyldopa and levodopa, might be expected to have decreased blood concentrations in the elderly. Increased bioavailability of levodopa, however, has been noted in elderly patients with Parkinson's disease. This is possibly due to reduced metabolism in the gut wall, and the effect may not occur when preparations containing a dopa decarboxylase inhibitor are prescribed—for instance, levodopa+acarbidopa (Sinemet).

DRUG-DRUG INTERACTIONS

Drug interactions affecting absorption may be due to a direct reaction between the drugs within the bowel lumen or to the effect of one of the drugs on bowel function—for instance, altered motility. The former type may be reduced by administering the drugs at different times.

Many interactions have been reported, but the problem is to assess their clinical importance. In many examples at least one of the interacting drugs is either not commonly used or could be replaced by a more rational choice of treatment. Cholestyramine binds to several drugs and has been shown to reduce the absorption of warfarin and digoxin. Since both these drugs have a narrow therapeutic index, this is of clinical importance, but the scope for this interaction to occur is limited as cholestyramine is not commonly used. Another frequently quoted example is the chelation interaction between tetracyclines and iron or antacids. If these drugs are necessary in the same patient there should be at least two hours between their administration. Tetracyclines are commonly prescribed, but there is usually a more rational choice of antibiotic available.

An early study of interactions affecting bowel function has shown that metoclopramide lowers and propantheline increases serum digoxin concentrations in patients undergoing chronic treatment with a slow dissolving formulation of digoxin. It was later found, however, that these drugs had no appreciable effect on digoxin absorption when a standard (Lanoxin) or micronised formulation was used. This adds further weight to the need to use only one standard digoxin formulation for a more reliable clinical response. The time to peak plasma concentration of lithium carbonate is shortened by metoclopramide and lengthened by proprantheline, which may make the plasma concentration monitoring of lithium more difficult to interpret. Although propantheline is little used now, a wide variety of drugs with atropine-like actions—such as tricyclic antidepressants, phenothiazines, and disopyramide—may produce similar effects through delayed gastric emptying. Antibiotics such as ampicillin may interfere with the enterohepatic circulation of oestrogens by altering the gut bacterial flora, and the decreased plasma oestrogen concentration could result in contraceptive failure. Care should always be taken when drugs are administered concurrently, but clinically important interactions are more likely to result from mechanisms other than changes in absorption.

PARENTERAL ADMINISTRATION

It is a general impression that intramuscular injection will lead to a more rapid onset of drug action. Although this is usually the case, it does not apply to all drugs. Phenytoin is slowly and irregularly absorbed after intramuscular injection, which leads to difficulty in achieving satisfactory control of seizures. Also the delayed absorption may lead to toxicity after change to the oral route. If it is impossible to give the drug by mouth then slow intravenous administration is more reliable. Diazepam is also better absorbed when ingested, unless care is taken to ensure a deep intramuscular injection. If there is decreased peripheral circulation the intramuscular and subcutaneous routes are not satisfactory sites for drug administration.

CONCLUSION

In conclusion many interacting factors will contribute to inter-individual differences in drug absorption. Mostly these affect the *rate* but not the *extent* of absorption and are therefore important only when an immediate therapeutic effect is required. When pronounced inter-individual differences in therapeutic response have been noted, these have been mainly attributed to differences in metabolism or excretion, rather than absorption.

Adverse drug interactions

JEFFREY K ARONSON, DAVID G GRAHAME-SMITH

In this chapter we shall discuss the incidence and mechanisms of adverse drug interactions, give examples of clinically important interactions, and mention other sources of information. We shall not discuss beneficial interactions.

In considering the incidence of adverse interactions we must distinguish between potential interactions—that is, the concurrent prescription of two drugs known to interact—and interactions that result in clinically obvious adverse effects. In one study[1] of 2422 patients studied prospectively during two months 113 (4.7%) were taking drugs with the potential for interaction but in only seven cases was there any clinical evidence of interaction (0.3% of all the patients; 6·2% of those potentially affected). With certain combinations of drugs, however, clinically important effects may occur more often. For example, in one survey of 1554 prescriptions for potassium chloride and 245 for spironolactone[2] 104 prescriptions were issued for the combination of those two (6·1%), and in a sample of 25 patients taking such a combination three developed hyperkalaemia (0·7% of all patients; 12% of those taking the combination). In a study of the use of oral anticoagulants[3] in 277 patients 94 were receiving other drugs that might have interacted (33·9%), and clinically significant interactions were thought to have occurred in six (2·2% of all patients; 6·4% of those taking combinations).

Unfortunately, there are problems in collecting incidence figures of this type. For example, it may often be difficult to determine whether an adverse effect of a drug occurs as a result of a drug interaction rather than as a result of, say, misuse of the drug or of an interaction between the drug and some peculiarity of the patient, such as renal or hepatic dysfunction. What is certain, however, is that the chance of an adverse drug interaction increases with the number of drugs the patient is taking.[4]

Most drug interactions concern only two drugs, although there are published examples of interactions among more than two drugs. In general, when two drugs interact one *precipitates* the interaction by one or more of several different mechanisms (see below) while the other is the *object* of the interaction, and its effects are either increased or reduced. We propose, therefore, for ease of discussion, that the drug that precipitates the interaction be called the *precipitant* drug while that whose effect is altered be called the *object* drug. Occasionally, two drugs may each alter the effects of the other (as in the complex interaction of phenytoin with phenobarbitone). In these few cases our proposed terms lose their significance.

Adverse drug interactions

The drugs most likely to be the object drugs in adverse interactions are those that have a steep dose-response curve—that is, drugs for which a small change in dose results in a relatively large change in effect, important in interactions causing decreased efficacy of the object drug; and those that have a low toxic:therapeutic ratio—that is, drugs for which the dose at which toxic effects start to occur is very little more than the therapeutic dose, important in interactions causing toxic effects of the object drug. Drugs fulfilling these criteria include anticoagulants, hypoglycaemics, anticonvulsants, antiarrhythmics and cardiac glycosides, drugs acting on the central nervous system, oral contraceptives, and antihypertensives. Those drugs most likely to be precipitant drugs may often be predicted on the basis of the various mechanisms of interaction—for example, drugs that are highly protein-bound (for example, sulphonamides, salicylates); alter hepatic metabolism either by stimulation (for example, phenytoin) or inhibition (for example, metronidazole, cimetidine); or have effects that either mimic that of the object drug (for example, central nervous depressants) or have some effect that interacts with an effect of the object drug (for example, aspirin, which causes gastric erosions and diminishes platelet aggregability, both of which increase the chance of gastrointestinal bleeding in patients taking oral anticoagulants).

The types of drug interactions are pharmaceutical, pharmacokinetic, and pharmacodynamic.

PHARMACEUTICAL INTERACTIONS

We have not hitherto considered those interactions that may be termed "pharmaceutical"—that is, those of a drug either with another drug in the same infusion solution or with the infusion solution itself. Interactions between drugs and infusion (saline or dextrose) solutions often take the form of loss of activity of the drug because of instability in solution. Table I lists the most important examples. Interactions between drugs and infusion solutions other than saline or dextrose are often due to other mechanisms[5] and may be avoided by avoiding such solutions for drug infusion. Interactions between two drugs in solution are far too numerous for individual discussion. In one study[6] of 67 different drugs all 2211 possible combinations of any two drugs were studied in both 0·9% saline (pH 7) and 5% dextrose (pH 4·3). Only effects that were visible after three hours (precipitation, turbidity, or colour change) were studied. Only 23 of the 67 drugs gave no visible positive results in all combinations and in one in 30 cases there was visible precipitation. Such interactions should be avoidable, and the following principles should be followed.

(*a*) Read the manufacturer's publications for specific warnings and to check that the drug is suitable for intravenous administration.

TABLE I—*Stability of some drugs in saline and dextrose solutions*

Unstable—infuse within 2 hours
Ampicillin
Stable for 6–8 hours
Frusemide
Benzylpenicillin
Diazepam
Stable for 12 hours
Flucloxacillin
Oxytetracycline
Tetracycline
Light-sensitive
Nitroprusside
Amphotericin B

(*b*) Give intravenous drugs by bolus injection whenever possible.

(*c*) Never use infusion solutions other than dextrose or saline for drug infusion.

(*d*) Avoid mixing drugs in the same infusion solution unless you know the mixture to be safe—for instance, potassium chloride and insulin.

(*e*) Mix the drug thoroughly in the infusion solution and check soon after and later during infusion for visible changes (turbidity, precipitation, colour change). Absence of such changes does not, however, guarantee the absence of an interaction.

(*f*) Prepare solutions only when needed (exceptions to this rule include drugs that are available in prepacked infusion solutions, such as KCl, lignocaine, metronidazole, chlormethiazole.)

(*g*) Label all infusion bottles clearly with the name and dose of drug added and the times of starting and ending the infusion.

(*h*) Use two separate infusion sites if it is necessary to infuse two drugs simultaneously unless it is known that there is no interaction.

(*j*) Consult your local hospital pharmacist if in doubt.

Other points are discussed in the 1976 DHSS report on this matter,[7] and extensive lists of potential interactions are given by Riley[6] and Grayson.[8]

PHARMACOKINETIC INTERACTIONS

By pharmacokinetic interactions we mean those interactions in which the disposition of the object drug is altered in some way by the precipitant drug. Such interactions are best considered according to which facet of drug disposition is affected.

Adverse drug interactions

Absorption

Although there are several mechanisms whereby the absorption of a drug may be altered by another drug—for example, the decrease in gastrointestinal motility caused by morphine-like drugs and anti-cholinergic drugs such as tricyclic antidepressants and chelation of calcium, aluminium, magnesium, and iron salts by tetracyclines—such effects are rarely of clinical importance. Exceptions are the interactions of cholestyramine with oral anticoagulants and digitoxin. Reduction of initial absorption and of reabsorption after biliary excretion increases requirements of the object drugs.

Protein binding

If a drug is highly protein bound (greater than 90%) in the plasma then displacement by a precipitant drug will result in a relatively large increase in the free concentration of object drug in the plasma and therefore to an increased effect. If the precipitant drug is withdrawn the reverse will occur. That the object drug must be highly protein bound is important—displacement of 5% of a drug that is 20% bound results in a change in free concentration from 80% to 85%, a negligible effect; on the other hand, a change in binding of 1% of a drug that is 99% bound (such as warfarin), leads to a change in free concentration from 1% to 2% of total, a doubling of the free concentration. That change is important, however, only if a large amount of the drug is in the plasma—if most of the drug is in the tissues even total displacement from plasma proteins will make little difference; hence only drugs with a low apparent volume of distribution (V_d) will be affected. The important drugs that fulfil these criteria for object drugs are oral anticoagulants, such as warfarin, bound 99%, V_d 9 l; oral hypoglycaemics, such as tolbutamide, bound 96%, V_d 10 l; and phenytoin, bound 90%, V_d 35 l. For the precipitant drug it is enough that it be highly protein bound to the same binding site as the object drug; the commonest precipitant drugs in such interactions are the sulphonamides, salicylates, derivatives of chloral (because of their metabolite trichloracetic acid), phenylbutazone, and oxyphenbutazone.

The importance of protein-binding-displacement interactions, however, has been exaggerated, and such interactions are usually of no clinical importance, The reason is that for drugs such as warfarin, phenytoin, and tolbutamide the total clearance rate is proportional to the fraction of drug unbound in the plasma, and after displacement of the object drug its rate of clearance from the body is increased. Thus at steady state the total concentration of drug in the plasma will have fallen to a new equilibrium value such that the free concentration is the same as it was before the introduction of the precipitant drug. In some cases the change in free concentration occurs so slowly that the compensatory increase in clearance reduces the transient increase in free concentration of the object drug to negligible proportions. Thus, provided the patient can "weather" the increase, if any, in free concentration of object drug for as long as it takes to reach a new steady state, such an interaction will not be of clinical importance. Indeed, only for warfarin has it been reported that such interactions may be important in causing adverse clinical effects, and those adverse effects may be avoidable by slow introduction of the precipitant drug. There is, however, another effect, important for phenytoin, in regard to the 'therapeutic" plasma concentration range. It is best discussed with an illustrative example. Suppose a patient has a therapeutically effective total plasma phenytoin concentration of 60 µmol/l ("therapeutic" range 40–80) of which 10% is free—that is the free concentration is 6 µmol/l. If the free fraction is doubled to 20% of total, although the free concentration at the new equilibrium will be, as before 6 µmol/l, it will represent 20% of the total concentration, which will have fallen to 30 µmol/l—that is, below the so-called "therapeutic" range. In fact for that patient the effective "therapeutic" range is lowered during the interaction.

Metabolism

If a drug is extensively metabolised it may become the object drug in an interaction if its metabolism by hepatic microsomal, or other, enzymes is either increased (enzyme induction) or inhibited by a precipitant drug. The precipitant drugs that commonly increase drug metabolism (enzyme inducers) are phenytoin, phenobarbitone, primidone, carbamazepine, rifampicin, griseofulvin, and alcohol (chronic use). Such interactions are of clinical importance. For example, an unwanted pregnancy may occur in patients taking oral contraceptive agents in the now conventional low-dose (oestrogen) preparations and an enzyme inducer. Warfarin metabolism may be increased by an enzyme inducer leading to higher dosage requirements; if the inducer is then withdrawn haemorrhagic complications may occur. Enzyme induction increases the hepatotoxic effects of paracetamol in overdose. The time course over which enzyme induction occurs is a few weeks.

Inhibition of hepatic microsomal enzymes may be caused by several drugs (metronidazole, phenylbutazone and oxyphenbutazone, chloramphenicol, isoniazid, cimetidine, and alcohol in acute intoxication) and the commonest object drugs are the oral anticoagulants and phenytoin. Some of the effects of inhibitors of warfarin metabolism are stereospecific—for example, phenylbutazone inhibits the metabolism of the S(−)enantiomer but induces the metabolism of the R(+) enantiomer; the overall effect on the racemic mixture is no apparent change in metabolism but since S(−)warfarin is more potent than R(+)warfarin the inhibitory effect predominates and a clinically important potentiation of warfarin effect occurs. Phenylbutazone interacts with warfarin in four other ways—directly by protein-binding displacement and indirectly by inhibition of platelet aggregation and by increasing the likelihood of gastrointestinal ulceration and thrombocytopenia. Also important are the interactions of phenytoin with isoniazid (in slow acetylators) and chloramphenicol, in which the effects of phenytoin are increased. Important examples of inhibition of *specific* metabolic processes include the interaction of monoamine oxidase inhibitors with tyramine-containing foods (such as cheese, red wine—tyramine metabolism by gut-wall monoamine oxidase is inhibited and hypertension results) and that of allopurinol with 6-mercaptopurine and azathioprine (whose metabolism is mediated by xanthine oxidase which is inhibited by alloxanthine, the active metabolite of allopurinol).

Active transport

Some drugs are transported by active systems that may be inhibited by a precipitant drug. A clinically important example is the effect of tricyclic antidepressants in blocking the transport of adrenergic neurone blockers (guanethidine, bethanidine, debrisoquine) to within nerve endings, thus attenuating their antihypertensive effects.

Excretion

Occasionally a precipitant drug may alter the urinary excretion of a compound that is excreted unchanged. An important example is the effect of quinidine in reducing digoxin excretion by the kidneys and thus increasing its plasma concentration (by, on average, a factor of two). The interaction, however, may also entail displacement from tissue-binding sites. Phenylbutazone reduces the renal clearance of chlorpropamide with a consequent increase in the risk of hypoglycaemia. Frusemide and ethacrynic acid decrease excretion of gentamicin, thus enhancing its potential for ototoxicity and nephrotoxicity; it is not known whether or not bumetanide has a similar effect.

PHARMACODYNAMIC INTERACTIONS

Pharmacodynamic interactions may be either direct or indirect.

Direct interactions

The most common direct pharmacodynamic interactions are those resulting from drugs acting on the central nervous system. Since most such drugs—for instance, benzodiazepines, alcohol, phenothiazines—have effects that result in the depression of central nervous function their concomitant use results in a combination of their separate effects. Other important examples of such additive effects are antihypertensive

TABLE II—*Some adverse drug interactions of clinical importance*

Object drug(s)	*Precipitant drug(s)*
Interactions in which effects of object drug are potentiated	
Acetohexamide	Phenylbutazone
Alcohol	CNS drugs, disulfiram, metronidazole
Amine-containing foods	Monoamine oxidase inhibitors
Amphetamines	CNS drugs, monoamine oxidase inhibitors
Azathioprine	Allopurinol
Beta-adrenoceptor blockers	Verapamil
Cardiac glycosides	Hypokalaemia (diuretics, purgatives, carbenoxolone, corticosteroids, amphotericin B), hypercalcaemia (vitamin C, calcium), quinidine
Cephaloridine	Potent diuretics (frusemide, ethacrynic acid)
Chlorpropamide	Phenylbutazone
CNS drugs	Other CNS drugs
Coumarin anticoagulants	Anabolic steroids, chloral hydrate, chloramphenicol, cimetidine, clofibrate, dextropropoxyphene, dipyridamole, disulfiram, D-thyroxine, indomethacin, mefenamic acid, metronidazole, oxyphenbutazone, phenylbutazone, salicylates, sulphinpyrazone, tetracyclines
Diuretics (potassium-sparing)	Diuretics (potassium-sparing), potassium chloride
Gentamicin	Potent diuretics (ethacrynic acid, frusemide)
Lithium	Diuretics (sodium-wasting)
Mercaptopurine	Allopurinol
Non-depolarising muscle relaxants	Aminoglycoside antibiotics, quinidine
Pethidine	Monoamine oxidase inhibitors
Phenytoin	Chloramphenicol, coumarin anticoagulants, disulfiram, isoniazid, phenylbutazone, sulthiame
Potassium chloride	Diuretics (potassium-sparing)
Tolbutamide	Chloramphenicol, clofibrate, coumarin anticoagulants, phenylbutazone, salicylates, sulphonamides
Verapamil	Beta-adrenoceptor blockers
Interactions in which effects of object drug are diminished	
Adrenergic neurone blockers (bethanidine, debrisoquine, guanethidine)	Chlorpromazine, tricyclic antidepressants
Antiarrhythmics	Hypokalaemia (diuretics, purgatives, carbenoxolone, corticosteroids, amphotericin B)
Carbenoxolone	Spironolactone
Cardiac glycosides (digitoxin)	Cholestyramine
Chlorpromazine	Barbiturates, orphenadrine
Cortisol	Barbiturates, phenylbutazone, phenytoin
Coumarin anticoagulants	Alcohol (chronic use), barbiturates, chloral hydrate, cholestyramine, cortisol, dichloralphenazone, diuretics, glutethimide, griseofulvin, nortriptyline, oestrogens, phenytoin, rifampicin
Oral contraceptives	Barbiturates, phenytoin, rifampicin
Oral hypoglycaemics	Diazoxide, diuretics
Phenytoin	Alcohol, barbiturates, carbamazepine
Tolbutamide	Rifampicin

CNS=Central nervous system.

drugs (which in combination may be harmful or beneficial) and the following combinations: frusemide (or ethacrynic acid) with gentamicin (ototoxicity); non-depolarising muscle relaxants with amino-glycoside antibiotics or quinidine (increased muscle relaxation); verapamil with propranolol (increased incidence of arrhythmias and possibly cardiac arrest); potassium-sparing diuretics either with each other or with potassium chloride (hyperkalaemia). An example of a more subtle potentiating interaction is that of warfarin with clofibrate, anabolic steroids, tetracyclines, or D-thyroxine (increased warfarin effect, possibly because of altered affinity of vitamin K for clotting factor receptors).

In passing it is worth while clearing up a misconception about the potentiating interactions of warfarin with some antibiotics. Such interactions are commonly attributed to the inhibitory effect of antibiotics on the gut flora responsible for synthesising vitamin K. Dietary vitamin K, however, will prevent a potentiation of warfarin effect even if vitamin K synthesis by gut flora (which in any case takes place mostly in the large bowel) is completely inhibited. Antibiotics such as chloramphenicol, metronidazole, and tetracycline, which do potentiate the action of warfarin, do so by other mechanisms. Thus, unless there is dietary deficiency of vitamin K, antibiotics such as those of the penicillin, cephalosporin, and aminoglycoside groups should be safe to use.

Interactions in which the precipitant drug antagonises the effects of the drug are common but are often beneficial—for instance, naloxone reversal of opiate effects, the treatment of poisoning with anticholinergic drugs using physostigmine. Important exceptions are the interaction of diuretics (thiazides or frusemide) or diazoxide with oral hypoglycaemic drugs (reduction in hypoglycaemic effects) and the attenuation of the therapeutic effects of carbenoxolone by spironolactone and of warfarin by oestrogens (increased clotting factor synthesis).

Indirect interactions

Indirect pharmacodynamic interactions are of two kinds. The first is the interaction in which the precipitant drug causes some alteration of fluid or electrolyte balance which influences the effect of the object drug. Important examples are: the enhancement of the effects of cardiac glycosides or the attenuation of the effects of antiarrhythmic drugs such as quinidine or lignocaine because of hypokalaemia secondary to diuretics; the attenuation of the effects of warfarin by diuretics in heart failure because of relief of hepatic congestion; and the increased retention of lithium due to sodium loss secondary to diuretics. This last example shows how a pharmacodynamic effect of a precipitant drug may cause a change in the pharmacokinetics of the object drug.

The second variety of indirect interaction results between oral anticoagulants and drugs that either cause gastrointestinal erosion or ulceration (such as non-steroidal anti-inflammatory drugs, corticosteroids) or decrease platelet aggregability (such as salicylates, phenylbutazone, and indomethacin). In such cases there will be either an increased tendency to bleed or, if bleeding occurs, impaired haemostasis.

SOURCES OF INFORMATION

We have not tried here to be comprehensive, but have aimed simply at discussing the basis of some of the commoner adverse drug interactions of clinical importance. One cannot, in any case, hope to remember all those interactions that might result in an adverse reaction, and a knowledge of sources of information is useful. We have listed in table II the most common interactions of clinical importance or possible importance. There are two other forms of more comprehensive listing available.

Textbooks

The following will be found helpful:

Drug Interactions and their Mechanisms by Ivan Stockley (published by the Pharmaceutical Press, London, and available from them at a give-away price).

Drug Interactions by P D Hansten (published by Lea and Febiger, Philadelphia).

Evaluations of Drug Interactions (published by the American Pharmaceutical Association, Washington DC).

Charts and slide-rules

The information contained in Stockley's monograph mentioned above has been brought up to date and summarised in the form of a wall chart, a pocket folder, and a cardboard slide-rule. They are available free from Boehringer Ingelheim, Berkshire. Alternatively there is an interaction disc based on the same slide-rule principle[9] (Medisc^{TM}) published by Excerpta Medica, but it may be difficult to obtain in Britain.

REFERENCES

1 Puckett WH, Visconti JA. An epidemiological study of the clinical significance of drug-drug interactions in a private community hospital. *Am J Hosp Pharm* 1971;**28**:247–53.

2 Simborg DW. Medication prescribing on a university medical service—the incidence of drug combinations with potential adverse interactions. *Johns Hopkins Med J* 1976;**139**:23–6.

3 Williams JRB, Griffin JP, Parkins A. Effect of concomitantly administered drugs on the control of long-term anticoagulant therapy. *Q J Med* 1976; NS**45**:63–73.

4 May FE, Stewart RB, Cluff LE. Drug interactions and multiple drug administration. *Clin Pharmacol Ther* 1977;**22**:322–8.

[5] Barrett CW. Drug stability and safety. *Pharmaceutical Journal* 1971;**206**:267.
[6] Riley BB. Incompatibilities in intravenous solution. *Journal of Hospital Pharmacy* 1970;**28**:228–40.
[7] Working party on the addition of drugs to intravenous infusion fluids. *Report.* London: DHSS, 1976. (Health Circular 1976; HC (76) 9.)
[8] Grayson JG. Incompatibilities of multiple additives to intravenous infusion fluids. *Pharmaceutical Journal* 1971;**206**:64–71.
[9] Whiting B, Goldberg A, Waldie PS. The drug disc: warning system for drug interactions. *Lancet* 1973;i: 1037–8.

Plasma protein binding of drugs

W E LINDUP, M C L'E ORME

Binding to plasma proteins is both a help and a hindrance to the distribution of a drug through the body. Transport in the bloodstream by binding to albumin helps a drug to reach regions remote from the site of administration. Because bound drug cannot readily leave the capillaries, however, the rate of distribution of drug into the tissues will be controlled by the concentration gradient produced by the concentration of unbound unionised drug. Usually, it is the unbound drug concentration that is considered to be pharmacologically and toxicologically active. The fraction of unbound drug can also influence the rate of drug elimination. Binding does, therefore, affect both the duration and intensity of drug action.

The binding and transport of endogenous and exogenous substances are two of several important functions of the plasma proteins (figure).

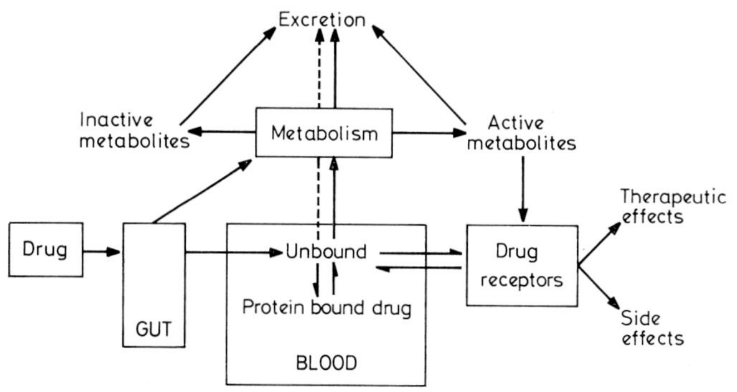

Protein binding and drug disposition

The endogenous substances include bilirubin, fatty acids, L-tryptophan, vitamins, and many hormones. Most drugs also bind to one or other of the plasma proteins, at least to some extent. Albumin is quantitatively the major binding protein for acidic and neutral drugs. Bases are bound to a lesser extent by albumin, and there is growing evidence that globulins are the major binding proteins for basic drugs.

Albumin has high affinity binding sites, which are probably specific for bilirubin and the fatty acids, but the high affinity sites for various hormones are located among the globulins. The binding of bilirubin serves a protective function in the newborn, where it prevents kernicterus by reduction of the diffusion of undue amounts of bilirubin into the brain. In a similar way the rate of diffusion of highly bound drugs into various tissues can be restricted.

There is no precise definition of a "highly" bound drug, but only when the percentage of a drug bound exceeds about 70% is binding likely to exert much influence on the distribution and pharmacokinetics of a drug. In the case of highly bound drugs—for instance, warfarin, carbenoxolone, or phenylbutazone—the unbound fraction may be considerably less than 1% of the total plasma drug concentration. The interaction of most drugs with the plasma proteins is a dynamic, reversible process with dissociation of bound drug molecules from the drug-protein complex occurring very rapidly, probably within milliseconds or less. The rate of dissociation of drug molecules from plasma proteins is therefore not a limiting factor in the uptake of drug from the bloodstream by major organs, whose perfusion time may be several seconds or more.

BINDING SITES

The drugs which tend to have the highest affinity for albumin are organic anions—for instance, carbenoxolone, phenylbutazone, warfarin—and they are also usually fairly lipid soluble. Quantitatively, binding to plasma proteins may be described by the law of mass action and analysed in terms of the number of binding sites (n) and the apparent association constant (K), a measure of affinity. These two binding constants combine to regulate the fraction of unbound drug available.

Isolated fractions of albumin and certain other plasma proteins have been available for several decades, and these are used for in-vitro experiments to determine values for n and K. These values can often give a reasonable prediction of the likely extent of binding to plasma proteins in vivo. In the case of many drug-albumin interactions there appear to be one or two primary (high affinity) binding sites available, together with a larger but variable number of secondary (lower affinity) sites.

Now that the overall structure of albumin is becoming clearer efforts are being made to locate and classify the binding sites. In addition to the separate and specific binding sites for bilirubin and the fatty acids, it appears there are at least two further separate sites which bind drugs. One site has been found to bind the benzodiazepines, various aromatic carboxylic acids, and L-tryptophan. Another site binds various anionic drugs such as warfarin, phenylbutazone, several sulphonamides, and other drugs. This type of work should eventually make the prediction of drug-drug displacement interactions easier and show whether the binding of endogenous substances is affected.

Albumin has been the most extensively studied of the binding proteins, but recent work has shown that α_1-acid glycoprotein (orosomucoid) is an important binding protein for basic drugs (table).

Drugs thought to interact with α_1-acid glycoprotein (orosomucoid)

Alprenolol	Imipramine
Chlorpromazine	Lignocaine
Dipyramidole	Propranolol
Disopyramide	Quinidine

BINDING AND DRUG DISPOSITION

Distribution

When drug distribution is complete—that is, at "steady-state" or equilibrium—the drug concentration throughout extracellular water will equal the unbound concentration in plasma. Cerebrospinal fluid, which contains little albumin, often reflects the concentration of unbound drug in plasma. The apparent volume of distribution of a drug (V_d) gives an indication of the extent of binding and distribution of a drug. The V_d of a highly bound drug, calculated from the total plasma concentration, is relatively small and for phenylbutazone it is about 0·1 l/kg. Extensive tissue binding results in the large volumes of distribution seen for drugs such as digoxin (6 l/kg) and chlorpromazine (20 l/kg).

Renal excretion

Protein-bound drug cannot undergo glomerular filtration and so only the unbound fraction can be filtered, which can prolong the half life of drugs that are neither actively secreted by the renal tubules nor rapidly metabolised. If an albumin-bound drug is subject to active renal excretion then binding is not usually a limiting factor. In fact, it tends to promote excretion by retaining drug in the bloodstream for delivery to the excretory system.

Hepatic elimination

As the result of earlier work, largely with the long-acting sulphonamides, a misconception has arisen that the long half life of a highly bound drug is solely the result of binding. There are numerous examples, however, of highly bound drugs and dyes that are rapidly metabolised and excreted. Furthermore, the half life of a given drug may vary widely among different species. There is therefore good reason to believe that the efficiency of the processes of elimination in the liver and kidney is of prime importance and that binding is a secondary factor.

If the processes of elimination (uptake and metabolism) are efficient then binding to plasma proteins acts as a delivery system. The rate of metabolism of some highly bound drugs such as propranolol depends on the rate of delivery to the liver via the bloodstream; this is called flow-dependent hepatic elimination. At the other extreme there are drugs—for instance, warfarin—where only the unbound fraction is taken up by the liver and with this flow-independent type of elimination binding serves primarily as a storage depot. Other drugs have elimination characteristics intermediate between these two extremes. Plasma clearance values for drugs are usually calculated from total drug concentrations, and the interpretation of these results should take into account the fraction bound.

FACTORS AFFECTING DRUG BINDING

The unbound fraction of drug present in plasma is dependent on the total concentrations of drug and albumin together with the values of n and K for the interaction. Any alteration in these binding constants, physiological or pathological in origin, will change the unbound fraction of drug.

Age is one physiological factor that may influence binding, and the unbound fraction appears to be higher in neonates and possibly in the elderly. There is, however, insufficient work on this topic to draw firm conclusions. Interindividual variations in the binding of basic drugs such as imipramine have been noted, and this may have a genetic basis. The presence of other drugs and the effects of disease are the two major factors that can affect binding.

Drug displacement

The binding of one drug can be inhibited by the presence of a second drug, and the mechanism may be either competitive, when drugs bind to the same site, or non-competitive, with the inhibitory drug causing a conformational change in the albumin molecule that inhibits the binding of the first drug. The inhibition of binding is probably mutual in many cases but it is usually only an increase in unbound fraction of one of the drugs that is of interest. Drug-displacement interactions are complex phenomena, and comparison of the relative affinities of two drugs for albumin does not offer an easy way to predict displacement. The drug acting as a displacing agent usually has to be present in fairly high concentration, as well as have a high affinity for albumin, to cause appreciable inhibition of binding. The non-steroidal anti-inflammatory drugs are a typical group of displacing agents. Intravenous heparin inhibits binding indirectly by raising the plasma concentration of fatty acids, which are potent binding inhibitors.

An increase in unbound drug concentration results in redistribution of drug from the plasma to other parts of the body. The pharmacological effect is likely to be enhanced, and there will be increased elimination of drugs excreted by glomerular filtration. If the drug is removed by flow-dependent elimination processes in the liver and kidney, displacement may cause a short-lived increase in half-life because the displaced drug diffuses to more remote sites and less drug is transported to the sites of elimination. The clinical implications of displacement interactions for the fetus have not yet been explored, but studies in animals have shown that this type of interaction can appreciably increase the amount of drug reaching the fetus.

The pharmacokinetics of drug displacement interactions and their consequences are complicated and have still to be fully elucidated. Koch-Weser and Sellers[1] give a more detailed but non-mathematical discussion. In general, the extent of enhancement of pharmacological activity depends on several factors: the degree of displacement, the speed of the pharmacological response, and the effect of displacement on the rate of elimination of the drug. The potentiation of pharmacological activity is transient and fades as a new steady state is established during co-administration of the drugs. In clinical practice this potentiation may well be missed and may not present a serious hazard.

Experience has shown, however, that pairs of drugs which interact in relation to drug binding sites on plasma proteins also interact at sites of metabolism and excretion. Two examples of clinically important interactions affecting drug displacement concern warfarin and tolbutamide. Both are displaced by phenylbutazone and several other drugs, and in both cases inhibition of hepatic metabolism by the displacing drug is a major feature of the interaction. Drugs likely to be implicated in clinically important displacement interactions will be highly bound to albumin and have a small apparent volume of distribution and therapeutic index.

Disease

Several diseases affect drug binding, and the usual result is an increase in the unbound fraction. Disease may also affect metabolism and excretion, a situation similar to many displacement interactions. The effect of disease on albumin may be either quantitative or qualitative or both.

Hypoalbuminaemia, as a result of injury or disease, will increase the unbound fraction of drug. Adverse reactions to phenytoin and prednisone, for example, are more common in patients with hypoalbuminaemia. In patients with renal insufficiency the binding of acidic and neutral drugs to albumin is inhibited by accumulated endogenous metabolites and possibly also by the changes in the structure of albumin. The binding of a variety of drugs is also decreased by liver disease, mainly as a result of hypoalbuminaemia, but accumulated endogenous metabolites—for instance, bilirubin—may contribute.

Plasma protein binding of drugs

In rheumatoid arthritis and other inflammatory conditions, when the albumin concentration is lowered, there will be a concomitant decrease in the binding of albumin-bound drugs. There is often, however, a considerable increase in the concentration of several globulins including α_1-acid glycoprotein (orosomucoid). Basic drugs such as propranolol are bound to this protein, and a considerable increase in the fraction of bound drug occurs in these circumstances.

THERAPEUTIC DRUG MONITORING

When the unbound fraction of drug is increased because of disease or other drugs the peak of unbound drug concentration during each dosage interval is higher than normal. The mean total drug concentration will be decreased so that the concentration of unbound drug will be within the usual range. Measurement of total drug concentration then would give the misleading idea that an increase in dosage was necessary to raise the total drug concentration into the therapeutic range. This would be potentially hazardous. In cases where inhibition of drug binding is suspected, measurement of the unbound drug concentration would be a better guide to treatment, but there are practical difficulties.

Methods for investigating drug binding to plasma proteins are too numerous to discuss here, but the most suitable in-vitro experimental methods are equilibrium dialysis, ultracentrifugation, and ultrafiltration. The concentration of drug in saliva or the erythrocyte/plasma drug concentration ratio may give a useful measure of in-vivo binding of selected drugs—for example, phenytoin. Unfortunately, none of these methods is suitable for large-scale routine use at present.

REFERENCES

[1] Koch-Weser J, Sellers EM. Binding of drugs to serum albumin (two parts). *N Engl J Med* 1976;**294**:311–6, 526–31.

FURTHER READING

Jusko WJ, Gretch M. Plasma and tissue protein binding of drugs in pharmacokinetics. *Drug Metab Rev* 1976;**5**:43–140.

Lindup WE. Drug-albumin binding. *Biochem Soc Trans* 1975;**3**:635–40.

Lindup WE. Methods for the measurement of drug binding to plasma proteins. In: Rietbrock N, Woodcock BG, Neuhaus G, eds. *Methods in clinical pharmacology*. Wiesbaden: Vieweg, 1980:267–73.

Sjöqvist F, Borga O, Orme M L'E. Fundamentals of clinical pharmacology. In: Avery GS, ed. *Drug treatment*. London: Churchill Livingstone, 1980: 1–61.

Elimination of drugs

H E BARBER, J C PETRIE

This chapter outlines the principles of drug elimination, principally by the liver and kidneys. Most elimination processes of drugs follow first-order elimination kinetics. In such processes a defined and constant fraction of a drug—for example, half—is irreversibly eliminated in a constant time. The half-life time ($t\frac{1}{2}$) in such first-order processes is the time taken for the concentration of the drug to fall to half its previous value, regardless of the initial concentration of the drug. Some drugs—for example, ethyl alcohol—follow zero-order elimination kinetics. In these processes elimination of the drug occurs at a constant rate, because the enzymes responsible for metabolism of drugs, and the active excretion processes, particularly in the kidney, become saturated.

DRUG CLEARANCE

Total drug clearance is the sum of the drug elimination processes. These include renal, hepatobiliary, faecal, pulmonary, and dermal. Secretions also contribute to the elimination of drugs—for example, in saliva and milk. Clearance is defined as the volume of the body compartment from which drug is removed in unit time. Drug clearance is usually a more useful indicator of the efficiency of the elimination process of a drug than the $t\frac{1}{2}$, because the latter may be a poor index for some drugs and may even be misleading because it depends on the volume of distribution of the drug. An illustrative analogy is two buckets of unequal sizes, each filled with water, with equal outlet holes at their bases. The water escapes under the influence of gravity with equal amounts of water being lost from each bucket. If the experiment is repeated, but equal amounts of drug are dissolved in both the large and small bucket, the clearance of the drug will be the same from both the large and small bucket. The $t\frac{1}{2}$ will not be the same, however, being longer for the larger bucket because the $t\frac{1}{2}$ relates to the capacity of the bucket (analogous to the volume of distribution of the drug) and inversely to the clearance.

The apparent volume of distribution (V_d) is the theoretical volume of the body compartments required to contain the amount of drug if it were uniformly distributed throughout the body in the same concentration as it is present in the blood. It should be understood that such compartments do not usually relate to recognised anatomical body spaces. Reversible distribution of drugs, as discussed in earlier chapter in this book, is influenced by the lipid solubility of the drug. The more lipid soluble the drug is, the more distribution into lipid compartments takes place and hence the larger is the V_d of the drug, thus affecting its elimination.

Drug clearance is also influenced by the rate of delivery of the drug to the organs of elimination, principally the liver and kidney, and by the capacity of the organs to eliminate the drug. In clinical practice most drugs are swallowed and with some, for example, propranolol, the bioavailability is low because only a fraction of the oral dose administered reaches the systemic circulation owing to extensive pre-systemic or first-pass elimination during absorption from the gut and passage through the liver. A drug such as propranolol is said to be subject to high hepatic intrinsic clearance and, therefore, has a high extraction ratio. If the intrinsic clearance is high the rate-limiting step in the elimination of the drug is hepatic blood flow. Such elimination is described as blood-flow limited or non-restrictive. Examples of other drugs concerned in such elimination include lignocaine, labetalol, metoprolol, chlormethiazole, morphine, pentazocine, and pethidine. An example of a drug subject to high renal clearance is para-amino hippuric acid, which has long been used to measure renal plasma flow. For drugs with high clearance values, whether given by mouth or intravenously, drug binding to plasma or tissue proteins does not greatly influence elimination of the drug because rapid dissociation of bound drug occurs, allowing elimination of both unbound and bound drug.

If the capacity of the organ of elimination to remove drugs is low, the removal process is the rate-limiting step and such elimination is capacity-limited or restrictive. For such drugs hepatic clearance depends on the concentration of free drug available to the elimination process, which depends on the extent of drug-protein binding but not on blood flow. Many drugs concerned in capacity-limited processes are bound to plasma albumin—for example, warfarin, phenytoin, diazepam, and tolbutamide. Reduction in the degree of protein binding of such drugs does not result in a change in steady-state concentration of free drug because any transient increase in free unbound drug, as a result of displacement from protein-binding sites, increases its availability for elimination. A reduction in drug-protein binding, however, leads to reduced steady-state total drug concentration and this could mislead the clinician, as has been shown in the example of the anticonvulsant drug phenytoin, which was administered to hypoalbuminaemic and control patients. The concentration of free drug was similar in the two groups, but the total concentration in the hypoalbuminaemic group was half that of the control group. Since it is the concentration of free drug that relates to pharmacological effect, and not of total drug (the concentration usually measured by routine hospital laboratories), unnecessary alterations in dosage based on the total concentration of drug in the blood, with predictable resultant toxicity, should be avoided. In general a clinically relevant drug-drug or drug-host interaction is unlikely to occur as a result of alterations in drug protein-binding unless free drug clearance is reduced because of reduced capacity for clearance by the organs of elimination together with increased free drug concentrations occurring because of reduced binding to proteins.

Renal excretion is the net effect of glomerular filtration, renal tubular reabsorption and secretion.

The glomerulus produces an ultrafiltrate, and only free drug is filtered. The glomerular filtration rate is roughly 10% of renal blood flow and when reduced by renal malfunction may lead to delayed excretion of drugs and their metabolites. This subject has been reviewed recently.[1]

When reabsorption is by passive diffusion, the pH of the dilute tubular urine is important, for this determines the relative proportions of ionised and unionised drug present, the latter being reabsorbed by diffusion. This principle has been made use of in forced diuresis: if the increased urinary flow rate achieved is combined with a judicious manipulation of pH of the tubular urine, increased drug elimination may be achieved. Thus forced alkaline diuresis which allows for an acidic drug to be in its ionised form promotes the excretion of drugs such as phenobarbitone and salicylate, whereas amphetamine excretion is enhanced in an acidic environment. Such forced diuretic procedures are inefficient and of little value when the amount of drug eliminated per unit time is a small fraction of the total in the body—for example, with digoxin; they are not of benefit where drugs are more efficiently eliminated by metabolism—for example, most barbiturates, tricyclic antidepressants, and the benzodiazepines.

If reabsorption is by carrier transport then competition for the transport site will allow more drug to be eliminated. This is seen in the action of uricosuric agents on urate reabsorption and also the action of diuretics in promoting the excretion of sodium and chloride.

The main site of tubular secretion of drugs is the proximal convoluted tubule. Secretion is via an acidic or basic pump mechanism having the characteristics of active transport. Thus organic acids such as urate and penicillin and the end products of metabolism—the glucuronides and sulphates—participate in the acid pump while bases like choline and histamine are transported by the other route. Competition for the transport sites may not occur between the acid and base carriers but competition within the sites can take place. The often quoted example of the reduced elimination of penicillin in the presence of probenecid is an example of this. The active transports are very efficient, and for highly cleared drugs may eliminate the bound form of the drug, as discussed earlier. This is seen in the case of penicillin G where roughly 90% of the antibiotic eliminated is by secretion, which proves a more efficient process than glomerular filtration.

Elimination of drugs

CONCLUSION

We have outlined some of the drug factors and principles underlying the elimination of drugs. Patient factors have not been discussed, but they also greatly influence drug clearance. Modification of dosages has been suggested for many drugs in patients with renal insufficiency[1] and at the extremes of age.[2 3] Although studies with model drugs, such as propranolol, have been reported in patients with hepatic cirrhosis[4 5] and thyrotoxicosis,[6] the influence on the clearance of many commonly used drugs and of other diseases and patient factors, such as the effect of additional concurrent medication, remains to be clearly established.

REFERENCES

1 Fabre J, Fox HM, Dayer P, Balant L. Differences in kinetic properties of drugs: implications as to the selection of a particular drug for use in patients with renal failure. *Clin Pharmacokinet* 1980;**5**:441–64.

2 Morselli PL, Franco-Morselli R, Bossi L. Clinical pharmacokinetics in newborn and infants. *Clin Pharmacokinet* 1980;**5**:485–527.

3 Vestal RE. Drug use in the elderly. A review of problems and special considerations. *Drugs* 1978;**16**:358–82.

4 Wood AJJ, Kornhauser DM, Wilkinson GR, Shand DG, Branch RA. The influence of cirrhosis on steady-state blood concentrations of unbound propranolol after oral administration. *Clin Pharmacokinet* 1978;**3**:478–87.

5 Williams RL, Mamelok RD. Hepatic disease and drug pharmacokinetics. *Clin Pharmacokinet* 1980;**5**:528–47.

6 Riddell JG, Neill JD, Kelly JG, McDevitt DG. Effects of thyroid dysfunction on propranolol kinetics. *Clin Pharmacol Ther* 1980;**28**:565–74.

Adverse reactions to drugs

MICHAEL D RAWLINS

Adverse drug reactions (defined as unintended effects of substances used in the prevention, diagnosis, or treatment of disease) are common. They are responsible for 3-5% of hospital admissions, occur in 10–20% of hospital inpatients, and have recently been reported in 40% of patients receiving drugs in general practice.[1]

Thompson and I[2] have suggested that adverse reactions and interactions can usually be logically and clinically divided (see table I) into those that form part of a drug's *normal* pharmacological actions (type A: augmented) and those that represent a *novel* response (type B: bizarre).

TABLE I—*Classification of adverse drug reactions*

Features	Type A	Type B
Pharmacology	Augmented	Bizarre
Predictable	Yes	No
Dose-dependent	Yes	No
Morbidity	High	Low
Mortality	Low	High

TYPE A (AUGMENTED) REACTIONS

Type A reactions (table I) are the results of qualitatively normal, but quantitatively abnormal, pharmacological effects of drugs. They may be due not only to the primary (or intended) pharmacological property of a compound, but also to its other effects—for instance, the anticholinergic actions of tricyclic antidepressants causing tachycardia, dryness of the mouth, and blurring of vision. Such reactions are usually predictable and dose-dependent; and, although they may be common, they are rarely life-threatening.

Type A reactions occur in individuals lying at the extremes of dose-response curves for pharmacological effects. Individuals at one end will show frank toxicity, while those at the other will be therapeutic failures (a form of adverse reaction). There are three causes for this type of response.

Pharmaceutical

Differences in pharmaceutical formulation can give rise to substantial alterations in the quantity of drug that is "available" to reach its site of action. As a consequence, most Western countries (including Britain) now have strict regulations governing drug content, release rate, and bioavailability. New formulations are carefully scrutinised by regulatory authorities—for example, the Committee on Safety of Medicines—and claims by pharmaceutical companies that their branded products are superior to cheaper generic equivalents are now unfounded.

Pharmacokinetic

Individual differences in absorption, distribution, and elimination result in differences in drug concentrations at the site of action. Enhanced absorption, or impaired elimination, cause an increase in plasma and tissue concentrations and may precipitate type A toxicity. Conversely, impaired absorption or accelerated elimination may result in therapeutic failure. Pharmacokinetic variability is therefore an important and common cause of type A reactions.

Bioavailability—the fraction of an oral dose reaching the systemic circulation—is determined not only by the extent of absorption across the gut wall, but also by the extent of "presystemic" (also called "first-pass") metabolism in the gut wall and liver during the absorptive period.[3] Variability in gastrointestinal absorption may also occur as a result of altered motility or in mucosal disease.[4] Variability in presystemic metabolism occurs with tricyclic antidepressants, some opiates, and neuroleptics (table II), and with many beta-adrenoceptor blockers (table III). With such drugs, type A reactions will occur commonly unless their dosages are carefully tailored to individual responses.

The most common pharmacokinetic cause for type A reactions is variability in the rate of elimination. The elimination of drugs excreted

TABLE II—*Adverse reactions to drugs acting on the central nervous system*

Group	Type A	Type B
Anticonvulsants*	Sedation, ataxia, enzyme induction	Pseudolymphoma,† rashes, porphyria
Antidepressants	Sedation, anticholinergic effects, sensitivity to pressor amines	Hepatotoxicity
Anxiolytics/ hypnotics	Sedation, withdrawal effects	Hepatotoxicity‡
Levodopa	Nausea, vomiting, dyskinesia, psychoses	Haemolytic anaemia
Opiates	Sedation, confusion, nausea, vomiting, respiratory depression	
Neuroleptics	Sedation, confusion, extrapyramidal reactions, hypotension, tardive dyskinesia	Hepatotoxicity§

* Phenytoin, phenobarbitone, carbamazepine.
† Phenytoin.
‡ Especially chlordiazepoxide.
§ Especially chlorpromazine.

unchanged by the kidney is directly proportional to renal function.[5] Patients with impaired renal function (including the elderly) are therefore particularly apt to develop type A reactions when given doses designed for healthy young adults. This especially includes digoxin and atenolol (table III), aminoglycosides (table IV), and cimetidine (table V). Adverse effects to these drugs can largely be avoided if their dosages are tailored to individuals' renal function. Many drugs are eliminated by metabolism to inactive products that are then excreted. Two common pathways of biotransformation—microsomal oxidation and acetylation—vary widely in their rate of metabolism. Individual differences are due to both genetic and environmental influences,[6 7] and are compounded by liver disease and (in some instances) cardiac and renal failure. Drugs undergoing elimination primarily by microsomal oxidation included anticonvulsants, antidepressants, most anxiolytics/hypnotics, and most neuroleptics (table II); some beta-adrenoceptor antagonists, oral anticoagulants, and theophylline (table III); some oral hypoglycaemics (table VI); and some non-steroidal anti-inflammatory drugs and H_1-antagonists (table V). For all these drugs, variability among patients is so great that it is now unacceptable to prescribe "fixed" or "standard" doses on a chronic basis without adjustments tailored to individual responses. For some drugs, the use of plasma concentrations to monitor treatment can also make an important contribution in preventing toxicity, and this may be expected to become increasingly important in the future.

TABLE III—*Adverse effects of cardiovascular drugs and respiratory drugs*

Group	Type A	Type B
Beta-adrenoceptor agonists	Tachycardia, tremor	
Beta-antagonists	Bradycardia, hypotension, heart failure, bronchospasm	Rashes, oculocutaneous syndrome*
Cardiac glycosides	Nausea, vomiting, arrhthmias	Gynaecomastia
Diuretics (potassium sparing)	Hyperkalaemia	
Inhaled steroids	Candidiasis, adrenal suppressions	
Methyldopa	Sedation, hypotension	Hepatotoxicity, fever
Oral anticoagulants	Haemorrhage, resistance	Rashes†
Theophylline	Nausea, vomiting, tachycardia	
Thiazide and loop diuretics	Hypokalaemia, gout	Vasculitis, thrombocytopenia

* Practolol.
† Phenindione, only rarely with warfarin.

TABLE IV—*Adverse reactions to some antimicrobial drugs*

Group	Type A	Type B
Aminoglycosides	Ototoxicity, nephrotoxicity*	Rashes
Cephalosporins	Nephrotoxicity*	Rashes
Isoniazid	Peripheral neuropathy	Hepatotoxicity
Penicillins	Diarrhoea, convulsions	Anaphylaxis, rashes
Sulphonamides	Diarrhoea, enzyme inhibition†	Agranulocytosis, rashes
Tetracyclines	Uraemia, tooth deformities	Photosensitivity,‡ Fanconi syndrome

* Especially in combination with frusemide.
† Sulphamethoxazole.
‡ Demethylchlortetracycline.

TABLE V—*Adverse reactions to miscellaneous drugs*

Group	Type A	Type B
Non-steroidal, anti-inflammatory	Gastric erosions, dyspepsia	Asthma, hepatotoxicity, bone marrow suppression
Paracetamol	Hepatotoxicity	Anaphylaxis
H_1 antagonists	Sedation, confusion	Photosensitivity
H_2 antagonists	Confusion, enzyme inhibition	
Topical steroids	Skin atrophy, rosacea, adrenal suppression	

Pharmacodynamic

Despite the importance of pharmacokinetic variability, at least part of the individual susceptibility to drugs is due to altered target organ sensitivity. Although this has been inadequately studied, both changes in receptors (density and affinity) and alterations in homoeostatic mechanisms are probably concerned. Altered target organ response accounts for much of the variation in response to warfarin[8] and for the rare condition of hereditary resistance.[9] Differences in oestrogen and progestogen receptor density appear to be a major determinant of the response to endocrine treatment in breast cancer.[10] A reduction in the gain of homoeostatic processes accounts for the precipitation of heart failure or bronchospasm with beta-antagonists (table II). Impaired homoeostasis in the elderly is a common cause of postural hypotension with neuroleptics (table II) and loop diuretics (table III), as well as hypothermia with many central nervous system depressant drugs.

The specific type A reactions shown in tables II to VI are those that are most often observed with commonly prescribed drugs. The drugs shown in table II are, with the exception of levodopa, central nervous system depressants (causing sedation, loss of concentration, and confusion), to which the elderly are particularly vulnerable. These adverse effects summate either when two (or more) of this group are prescribed together, or if the patient takes alcohol. Although tolerance to the central sedative effects of these drugs occurs, appropriate advice about driving, operating heavy machinery, or drinking should be given to patients who are starting treatment.

Alkylating cytotoxic drugs (table VI) are mutagenic, and many have been shown to be carcinogenic in animals. Some have been shown to be carcinogenic in man, and they probably all possess this feature. In treating malignant disease such risks are clearly justified, but the use of alkylating cytotoxic drugs for non-malignant conditions clearly warrants careful consideration.

TABLE VI—*Adverse reactions to drugs with metabolic and endocrine effects*

Group	Type A	Type B
Carbimazole	Myxoedema	Agranulocytosis
Cytotoxics	Bone-marrow suppression, carcinogenicity	
Insulin	Hypoglycaemia	Haemolytic anaemia
Oral contraceptives	Withdrawal bleeding, break-through bleeding, thromboembolism	Porphyria, hepatotoxicity
Oral hypoglycaemics	Hypoglycaemia	Alcohol flushing*

* Chlorpropamide.

All non-steroidal anti-inflammatory drugs produce dyspepsia and some loss of blood (usually slight) from the gastrointestinal tract. They may also cause acute gastric erosions. Whether these drugs produce peptic ulceration, or cause massive haemorrhage and perforation in pre-existing ulcers, is still disputed. Despite this, it it wiser to avoid such drugs in patients with known duodenal or gastric ulcers unless clinical circumstances suggest that the possible risk is outweighed by the likely benefits. Sedation and confusion are common adverse effects of H_1-antagonists; confusion may also occur with H_2-antagonists, particularly in the elderly and others with reduced renal function.

TYPE B (BIZARRE) REACTIONS

Type B reactions are bizarre, qualitatively abnormal (table I) effects, which are apparently unrelated to a drug's normal pharmacology. Again, there are three basic causes.

Pharmaceutical

Byproducts of chemical synthesis—for instance aspiryl anhydride—or in-vitro degradation products, such as tetracyclines and penicillins, may give rise to toxic effects that have no relation to a drug's known pharmacological properties. Similarly the additives, excipients, colorisers, and binders that make up a pharmaceutical product—for example, lactose, glutein, tartrazine—may themselves cause toxicity, or may react with the drug itself to yield toxic derivatives such as carboxymethylcellulose and penicillin.

Pharmacokinetic

Individual differences in the overall rate and extent of absorption, distribution, and elimination results in changes in the intensity of a drug's effects, which, as we have seen, are important causes of type A reactions. It is theoretically possible, however, that the toxicity of some compounds is mediated via the formation of unusual, or novel, metabolites. There is evidence that the hepatotoxicity of methyldopa and isoniazid (tables III and IV) may be due to this process. It has also been suggested that the formation of electrophilic drug metabolites, which can bind covalently to tissue macromolecules, may result in the production of complete antigens or autoantibodies,[11] but at present there is no convincing example of such a mechanism at work.

Pharmacodynamic

Some type B reactions are due to genetic abnormalities which result in altered target organ responses.[2] These include haemolysis with oxidant drugs—for instance, sulphonamides, 8-aminoquinolines—in individuals with red cell glucose-6-phosphate dehydrogenase deficiency or certain haemoglobinopathies; the precipitation of acute porphyria with enzyme-inducing agents; malignant hyperpyrexia with inhalational anaesthetics and muscle relaxants; and periodic paralysis with drugs that alter some potassium.

Many type B reactions in tables II–VI appear to have an immunological basis. Nevertheless, not all immunological reactions are of type B, for in those instances where a drug is antigenic per se—for instance, antisera, polypeptides—the development of immunological effects is predictably type A.

CONCLUSIONS

The "augmented-bizarre" classification of adverse reactions used in this chapter is intended to provide a logical framework to the understanding, diagnosis, and management of drug toxicity. In some instances it must be accepted that due to our ignorance of the pharmacology of certain drugs, some apparent type B reactions will in the future need reallocation. In clinical practice, however, most type A reactions are preventable by careful dosage titration; they produce a clinical picture that is an extension of their normal pharmacological actions; and they can usually be managed either by appropriate adjustment of the dosage, by substitution of a more selective agent, or by giving an additional drug to antagonise unwanted effects. In contrast, type B reactions are often (though not invariably) unpredictable and usually require complete withdrawal of the offending drug.

REFERENCES

[1] Davies DM. History and epidemiology. In: Davies DM, ed. *Textbook of adverse drug reactions*. Oxford: Oxford University Press, 1977:5-9.

[2] Rawlins MD, Thompson JW. Pathogenesis of adverse drug reactions. In: Davies DM, ed. *Textbook of adverse drug reactions*. Oxford: Oxford University Press, 1977:10-31.

[3] Routledge PA, Shand DG. Presystemic drug elimination. *Ann Rev Pharmacol* 1979;**19**:477-8.

[4] Parsons RL, David JA. Gastrointestinal disease and drug absorption. In: Prescott LF, Nimmo WS, eds. *Drug absorption*. Sydney: Adis Press, 1979:262-77.

[5] Smith SE, Rawlins MD. *Variability in human drug response*. London: Butterworth, 1973.

[6] Vesell ES. Gene-environment interactions in drug metabolism. In: Turner P, ed. *Clinical pharmacology and therapeutics*. London: Macmillan 1980:63-79. (Proceedings of the First World Conference.)

[7] Conney AH, Pantuck EJ, Pantuck CB, *et al*. Variability in human drug metabolism. In: Turner P, ed. *Clinical pharmacology and therapeutics*. London: Macmillan, 1980:51-62. (Proceedings of the First World Conference.)

[8] Routledge PA, Chapman PH, Davies DM, Rawlins MD. Pharmacokinetics and pharmacodynamics of warfarin at steady state. *Br J Clin Pharmacol* 1979;**8**:243-7.

[9] O'Reilly RA, Aggeler PM, Hoag MS, Leong LS, Kropatkin ML. Hereditary transmission of exceptional resistance to coumarin anticoagulant drugs. The first reported kindred. *N Engl J Med* 1964;**271**:809-11.

[10] McGuire WL, Horwitz KB, Pearson OH, Segeloff A. Current status of estrogen and progesterone receptors in breast cancer. *Cancer* 1977;**39**:2934.

[11] Assem ESK. Drug allergy. In: Davies DM, ed. *Textbook of adverse drug reactions*. Oxford: Oxford University Press, 1977:380-96.

Drugs in children

GEORGE RYLANCE

Children are not "little adults" but rather immature individuals whose bodies and organ functions are in a continuing state of development. More particularly, the newborn infant has to adapt very rapidly to a new environment by going through a series of rapid and continuous anatomical and physiological changes. It is not surprising, therefore, that the pharmacokinetics and toxicity of most drugs vary considerably throughout the paediatric age range and may differ profoundly from findings in adults.

DRUG ABSORPTION

The rate of drug absorption into the systemic circulation depends on both the route of administration and the drug's physicochemical properties—molecular weight, pKa, and lipid solubility. The latter primarily determine the rate and extent of a drug's passage across membranes and apply equally to all ages. Tissue perfusion is an important factor relating to the route of administration. There are no functional differences between the older infant, child, and adult that should affect gastrointestinal absorption, although the rate, but not extent, of absorption may be increased by using liquid preparations of many drugs, and these formulations are often preferred in the young child.

In the newborn period, and after the first day of life, gastric contents are less acidic, and the gastric emptying time and intestinal transit time are considerably slower than at any other age. Consequently, drugs such as penicillin G and ampicillin, which are partially inactivated by a slow pH, have greater overall absorption when swallowed.[1 2] The slow gastric emptying time reduces the absorption of some drugs, while others may achieve greater absorption because of prolonged contact with the bowel wall during the longer transit period through the intestine.

Absorption from intramuscular and subcutaneous sites depends mainly on tissue perfusion, and if this is adequate it is similar in children and adults. The vasomotor instability in the newborn period might theoretically cause delay in absorption from peripheral sites, although in practice the therapeutic effectiveness of drugs given via these routes suggests that this is not an important factor.

DRUG DISTRIBUTION AND PROTEIN BINDING

The distribution process regulates the amount of drug reaching specific body compartments or tissues and hence the concentration of the drug at the receptor site. It is mainly influenced by the tissue mass, fat content, blood flow, membrane permeability, and degree of protein binding.

The relative body fat content is lowest in the newborn, particularly in preterm and light-for-dates babies. Thereafter, the relative mass of subcutaneous tissue rises to a maximum at 9 months of age, decreases until 6 years, and subsequently increases towards adolescence. The relative proportions of body water compartments also vary with age. As a percentage of total body weight the total body water falls from 87% and 77% in the preterm and term newborn baby respectively to 73% at 3 months, 59% at 1 year, and 55% in the adult. Similarly, extracellular water falls from 45% of the total body weight in the term newborn infant to 33% at 3 months, 28% at 1 year, and 20% in the adult.[3] Most drugs are bound to intracellular components but in addition are distributed evenly throughout the total and extracellular body water and, to some extent, body fat. The variability with age in concentrations of water-soluble and fat-soluble drugs at the receptor sites arising from these changes in compartment volumes and resulting from similar weight-related drug doses are obvious.

In addition the blood-brain barrier appears to be more permeable in the newborn period and thereby allows increased passage of some drugs across it, a fact that may be advantageous in the antibacterial treatment of meningitis at this age.

Extracellular binding to plasma proteins depends on the amount of binding proteins and the drug affinity constant for proteins, and these are directly or indirectly modified by pathophysiological conditions and by other drugs and compounds. A quantitative and qualitative reduction in plasma protein binding occurs in the newborn period. At this stage, babies, and particularly preterm babies, have lower plasma albumin concentrations than at other ages (30–40 g/l), and the albumin is qualitatively different and has a lower affinity for drugs. Further modification of plasma protein binding by the higher free fatty acid and bilirubin concentrations and the lower blood pH is likely to occur at this age.[4]

Information on drug protein binding in older children is limited, but from indirect evidence of cerebrospinal fluid and saliva levels, similar degrees of binding have been observed for carbamazepine, phenobarbitone, and phenytoin.[5–7] An increase in the free drug allows greater availability for metabolism and excretion, and the net effect of change is not wholly predictable.

The few studies reporting drug volumes of distribution in children suggest that there is greater variability in these subjects, there being generally the greatest values in the newborn period, progressively reducing but remaining relatively greater than in adults through childhood until equivalence is reached in adolescence.

ELIMINATION

Elimination of a drug is effected by metabolism or excretion, or both, of the parent drug. Drug elimination rates vary considerably in the newborn, infants, older children, and adults.

Metabolism

The liver is quantitatively the most important organ for drug metabolism at all ages. The overall rate of metabolism probably depends on both the size of the liver and the metabolising ability of the appropriate microsomal enzyme system. Liver volume relative to body weight decreases from birth to adulthood, the relative volume in the first year of life being twice that at 14 years.[8] This may explain why rates of drug metabolism are greatest in late infancy and early toddlerhood and become progressively less rapid through childhood to adolescence and adulthood. In the newborn period the microsomal enzyme systems are immature, and at this time the relative contributions of hepatic size and immaturity of the enzyme system probably determine drug metabolising rates. For most drugs in this period the rates of elimination appear to be slower than in later childhood. In older children the microsomal enzyme system activity per unit volume of liver is similar to that in adults (G W Rylance *et al* at the annual meeting of the British Paediatric Association, York, 1980), although there is probably wide variability.

Excretion

The ultimate route of elimination of most drugs is via the kidney. Developmental changes affecting the glomerular filtration and tubular secretory excretion processes are therefore important. The former attains adult values per unit surface area from about 2½–5 months of age, but in the newborn period it is only 20–40% of that in adults.[10] Tubular secretory and reabsorptive mechanisms reach adult capacity by about 7 months.[9] Consequently, drugs excreted by glomerular filtration—for instance, digoxin and gentamicin—and those for which tubular secretion is important—for example, penicillin—are eliminated less rapidly in the newborn than in older infants and children.

The generally larger volumes of distribution and faster rates of elimination of drugs in children compared with adults necessitate the higher weight-related doses in order to reach similar plasma drug concentrations. Not only are there pronounced differences in kinetic values between children and adults, but there is pronounced variability among individuals in childhood, particularly in the younger age groups.

ADVERSE EFFECTS

The overall incidence of adverse drug reactions in children varies in published data from 6% to 17%[10 11] and is similar to that reported for adults.[12] A higher rate (24·5%) has been reported in newborn infants,[13] which may reflect the slower rates of drug elimination and the greater magnitude of drug exposure in the newborn period.

As in adults most reactions relate to the gastrointestinal tract, followed by the haematological, cutaneous, neurological, metabolic, cardiovascular, and respiratory systems.[11 12] In the newborn hypertension, cardiac arrhythmias, renal failure, gastrointestinal reactions, and hypoglycaemia are the most frequent moderate/major adverse reactions.[13]

DRUG INTERACTIONS

Most children given drugs in hospital receive more than one and drug-drug interactions therefore need to be considered in prescribing. Many of the known interactions reported from adult practice, however, concern drugs not commonly used in paediatric practice, such as warfarin and the oral hypoglycaemic agents. In children interactions involving anticonvulsant drugs, either with each other or with other drugs, are likely to be those most commonly seen.

Children often receive "over the counter" drugs for minor ailments, but the problems of interactions resulting from these medications are not known.

DRUG CONCENTRATION MONITORING

The indications for monitoring drug concentrations in body fluids are the same for children as adults. The practice, however, is likely to be of particular relevance in children for several reasons. Inter- and intra-individual variation in drug response in childhood is greater than at any other time, and titration of dose to the therapeutic response is unsuitable for most of the commonly prescribed drugs in children (antimicrobials, anticonvulsants, anti-inflammatory agents). In addition the therapeutic index of some drugs appears narrower in the young.

Nevertheless, few therapeutic ranges for drugs have been reported specifically in children, and if, as seems likely, there are pharmacodynamic differences for some drugs between children and adults, establishing relevant therapeutic ranges is mandatory. In most cases monitoring drug concentrations in blood is the most appropriate approach, but children generally dislike its invasive nature. The problem may be offset by using saliva as the body fluid for drug assay, although this considerably reduces the scope and possibly the accuracy of the drug monitoring.

The large fluctuation in blood or saliva concentrations between doses and possible contamination of saliva by drug retained in the mouth make interpretation of drug concentrations particularly difficult in children.

REFERENCES

1 Huang NN, High RH. Comparison of serum levels following the administration of oral and parenteral preparations of penicillin to infants and children of various age groups. *J Pediatr* 1958;**42**:567–8.
2 Silverio J, Poole JW. Serum concentrations of ampicillin in newborn infants after oral administration. *Pediatrics* 1973;**51**:578–80.
3 Friis-Hansen B. Body water compartments in children: Changes during growth and related changes in body composition. *Pediatrics* 1961;**28**:169–81.
4 Krasner J, Yaffe SJ. Drug-protein binding in the neonate. In: Morselli PL, Garrattini S, Sereni F, eds. *Basic and therapeutic aspects of perinatal pharmacology*. New York: Raven Press, 1975:357–66.
5 Rylance GW, Butcher GM, Moreland TA. Saliva carbamazepine levels in children. *Br Med J* 1977;i:1481.
6 Jalling B. Plasma and cerebrospinal fluid concentrations of phenobarbital in infants given single doses. *Dev Med Child Neurol* 1974;**16**:781–93.
7 Borofsky LG, Louis S, Kutt H. Diphenylhydantoin in children. Pharmacology and efficacy. *Neurology* 1973;**23**:967–72.
8 Rylance GW, Cowan MD, Moreland TA. Liver volume estimation in children. Proceedings of the Paediatric Research Society Meeting, Spring 1980. *Arch Dis Child* 1980;**50**:824.
9 West JR, Smith HW, Chasis H. Glomerular filtration rate, effective renal blood flow, and maximal tubular excretory capacity in infancy. *J Pediatr* 1948;**32**:10–8.
10 McKenzie MW, Stewart RB, Weis CF, Chuff LE. A pharmacist based study of the epidemiology of adverse drug reactions in paediatric medicine patients. *Am J Hosp Pharm* 1973;**30**:898–903.
11 Whyte J, Greenan E. Pattern and quality of recording pre-admission drug treatment in paediatric patients. *Br Med J* 1976;i:61–3.
12 Hurwitz N, Wade OL. Intensive hospital monitoring of adverse reactions to drugs. *Br Med J* 1969;i:531–6.
13 Aranda JV, Portuguez-Malvisi A, Collinge J, Outerbridge E. Adverse drug reactions (ADR) in the newborn intensive care unit. *Proceedings of the seventh international congress of pharmacology* 1978:2880. (Abstracts.)

Drugs and the elderly

LAWRENCE E RAMSAY, GEOFFREY T TUCKER

The risk of adverse reactions overshadows all other considerations when prescribing for the elderly, although there is some suggestion that general practitioners, who are responsible for the bulk of prescribing, may not be fully aware of this.[1] Elderly patients are more likely than the young to react adversely to drugs prescribed in hospital,[2] and they are also more likely to be admitted to hospital[3] or to die[4] because of adverse reactions. Note, however, that such studies do not display the other side of the coin—the benefits of drug treatment—nor can we assume that all adverse reactions are preventable. If the elderly have a genuine need for more drugs than the young, as seems probable, they will inevitably pay some price for effective treatment, even if prescribing was beyond reproach. In fact, most doctors will admit that prescribing (particularly that of other doctors) is less than perfect, and we should aim at reducing adverse effects in the elderly to the minimum while avoiding a harmful degree of nihilism.

The high incidence of adverse reactions in the elderly has two distinct components, each with its own remedy. One relates to the pattern of prescribing in the elderly, and might yield to changes in prescribing habits. The other reflects the propensity of older patients to react adversely to certain individual drugs, and might be countered by more informed use of these drugs.

PRESCRIBING IN THE ELDERLY

The elderly receive more drugs than the young. While those aged over 65 make up 12% of the population they account for 33% of the national expenditure on drugs.[5] In one general practice 87% of those aged 75 or over were having regular drug treatment, and no fewer than 44% were taking three or more drugs regularly.[6] In addition many of the conditions more prevalent in the elderly, such as heart failure and Parkinsonism, need treatment with drugs that have a narrow margin between therapeutic and toxic doses. On the other hand, the use of some drugs with a more favourable therapeutic ratio—for example, those for skin diseases—does not increase with age.[7] Thus the elderly receive more drugs, and are more likely to receive relatively toxic drugs, and this is entirely to be expected from the pattern of illness in the community. What is not known is how much of this prescribing is unnecessary, ineffective, or inappropriate. Indeed, we may never know, because the topic is extremely subjective and sensitive.[1] We suspect, however, that adverse effects in the elderly could be reduced considerably, without loss of therapeutic benefit, by a concerted effort to prescribe only drugs that are necessary and have proved to be effective and by a shift from relatively toxic drugs to safer alternatives. It is encouraging to note the large fall in the prescribing of barbiturates that resulted from just such a policy.

The polypharmacy that prevails in the elderly has further important consequences. *Drug interactions* are more likely, and can be avoided only by constant vigilance. Ideally all prescribing should be in the hands of a single doctor. If not, it is important for all communications between hospital and general practitioner (in either direction) to include a complete list of the drugs and doses prescribed. Comments from hospital doctors on *repeat prescribing*, and on the writing of prescriptions by ancillary staff, are seldom welcome, and these aspects are under examination within general practice.[1] As many as half of those aged over 70 obtain drugs on repeat prescriptions.[7] Cardiovascular and psychotropic drugs figure prominently in these scripts,[7] and are also important causes of adverse reactions in the elderly. Finally, *non-compliance* deserves mention, although cynics may argue that it is more often a protection against adverse reactions than the cause. Non-compliance is not a problem confined to the elderly,[8] but it tends to increase with the number of drugs (and doses) given, and treatment errors are certainly common. In one study half of the elderly patients discharged from hospital had deviated from their recommended treatment within 10 days.[9] Poor understanding seems more of a problem than deliberate non-compliance, and most readers will be familiar with the "Nitrazepam (Mogadon) 5 mg in the morning and Bendrofluazide (Neo-naclex) 5 mg at bedtime" type of mistake. Adherence to treatment can be helped by simple clear instructions, in writing if necessary, and by simplifying the regimen, and will certainly not be good if the patient cannot read the label, open the container, or swallow the tablets. Tear-off calendars or tablet identification cards can reduce mistakes[10] but are not widely used so far as we know. Compliance can be checked easily by a surprise raid on the medicine cupboard during a home visit. Supervision of treatment should be arranged if all else fails.

INCREASED ADVERSE REACTION RATE TO INDIVIDUAL DRUGS

The elderly are more likely to react adversely to a given dose of some drugs but not to others. Reports from the Boston Collaborative Drug Surveillance Program have shown that older patients react significantly more often to nitrazepam,[11] flurazepam,[12] diazepam,[13] chlordiazepoxide,[13] heparin,[14] and potassium chloride[15] but not to several other drugs including theophylline,[16] frusemide,[17] and methyldopa.[18] The possible causes for increased susceptibility of the elderly to certain drugs are as follows.

Altered pharmacokinetics

Current knowledge is summarised in table I, and was detailed in recent reviews.[19 20] As regards clinical relevance the important distinction is between those drugs eliminated largely by renal clearance and those that are metabolised. Renal function declines linearly from the age of 30, and the clearance of drugs eliminated largely by the kidney, whether by filtration or tubular secretion, is reduced to an important degree in old age. This matters little if the drug has a wide margin between therapeutic and toxic doses (penicillin, for example), but the elderly are distinctly at risk from the accumulation of drugs such as digoxin, lithium, and gentamicin unless the dose is lowered. The serum creatinine concentration is not an accurate reflection of renal function in the elderly, as creatinine production falls with age. Creatinine clearance must either be measured directly or be estimated from a nomogram using age, sex, body weight, and serum creatinine concentration.[21]

The pharmacokinetics of some drugs that are metabolised are altered in the elderly (table I), but unfortunately the main pattern to date has been one of inconsistency. The everyday observation that some 80 year olds are "good" and some 60 year olds "old" reflects a difference between biological and chronological aging, and this makes the elderly a remarkably heterogeneous group to study. In addition, the effects of aging per se have not been separated satisfactorily from environmental

TABLE I—*Changes in pharmacokinetics in the elderly*

Absorption	Unaltered
Distribution	
Body weight ↓	Increased dose per unit body weight
Body water ↓ Body fat ↑	Water soluble drugs have higher blood levels, lower distribution volume; lipid soluble drugs have lower blood levels, higher distribution volume
Plasma albumin ↓	Protein binding reduced (phenylbutazone, tolbutamide) or unaltered (diazepam, salicylate)
Metabolism	
Oxidation	Reduced for some drugs (chlormethiazole, phenylbutazone) but not others (diazepam, warfarin). "First pass" metabolism of chlormethiazole, propranolol reduced
Hydrolysis Reduction Conjugation	Unaltered so far as is known
Renal clearance	Glomerular filtration/tubular secretion decline with age
Environmental factors Smoking ↓ Caffeine ↓ Alcohol ↓ Altered diet	Reduced induction of hepatic microsomal enzymes. Enzymes may also be "resistant" to induction

TABLE II—*Drugs known to be common or serious causes of adverse reactions in the elderly*

Drug	Problem	Action
Benzodiazepines	Daytime drowsiness	Half dose
Tricyclic antidepressants	Drowsiness, postural hypotension, anticholinergic	Half dose
Phenothiazines*	Extrapyramidal reactions	Avoid if possible
Digoxin	Reduced clearance	Reduce dose; rarely needed in sinus rhythm
Phenylbutazone	Increase in all reactions, and in marrow aplasia	Short courses only; choose safer alternative
Tetracyclines†	Renal failure	Consider alternative
Antihypertensive drugs	Postural hypotension	Avoid bethanidine, guanethidine, debrisoquine
Anti-Parkinsonism drugs	Confusion, postural hypotension, anticholinergic	Consider hospital supervision
Oral hypoglycaemics	Nocturnal hypoglycaemia	Choose short-acting drug
Thyroxine	Myocardial ischaemia	Consider hospital supervision
Barbiturates	Many	Do not use
Opiates	Increased sensitivity	Reduce dose
Warfarin	Increased sensitivity	Reduce dose
Heparin	Bleeding	Use for 48 h only

* In addition to well-recognised drugs (chlorpromazine, promazine, thioridazine) phenothiazines are used for vertigo (for instance, prochlorperazine, (Stemetil)) and in combinations (for instance, fluphenazine in Motipress, Motival).
† Doxycycline does not appear to worsen renal failure.

influences, such as reduced cigarette smoking, altered diet, or living in an institution. For drugs that are metabolised there are at present no general rules of value to the prescriber.

Altered pharmacodynamics

It has been difficult to prove altered "sensitivity" of the elderly to a given concentration of drug at receptor sites, but there is now evidence that this is so for three drugs. Enhanced sensitivity to nitrazepam[22] and warfarin[23] is the probable reason for their increased toxicity (or reduced dose requirement) in the elderly. On the other hand, older patients are *less* sensitive to β-adrenergic blockers at the cellular level,[24] and they also have a smaller antihypertensive response than the young to β-blockers.[25]

Impaired homoeostasis is generally accepted as one reason why many drugs cause or worsen confusion, postural hypotension, hypothermia, or falls in the elderly. These phenomena have received little formal study, and the line between aging per se and early disease is not easily drawn.

Multiple disease states are common, and it is all too easy to overlook an important contraindication to a drug even when it has been documented before. Diagnoses get "lost" remarkably often in hospital notes and, we suspect, in general practitioners' records. The use of a comprehensive problem list, easily checked when a new drug is prescribed, has much to commend it. Inclusion in the list of previous adverse reactions should prevent the unforgivable error of causing the same side effect twice.

SAFE PRESCRIBING IN THE ELDERLY

In table II we make specific recommendations for several drugs, singled out because they are common or serious offenders in the elderly. Apart from this we can only reiterate some of the principles of sound prescribing, because they are particularly important to the elderly. Consider whether a drug is really needed, stick to drugs of proved efficacy, and be sceptical about new drugs. Check whether your chosen drug causes problems in the elderly, and use a safer alternative when possible. Check specifically for contraindications and potential interactions, and double check when using a combination product. Simplify treatment, and be sure that the patient understands it. Monitor the response, be alert to possible side effects, and discontinue the drug as soon as possible. Finally, and most important, always err on the side of *low doses* in the elderly.

REFERENCES

1 Knox JDE. Prescribing for the elderly in general practice. *J R Coll Gen Pract* 1980;**30**, suppl 1:1–8.

[2] Hurwitz N. Predisposing factors in adverse reactions to drugs. *Br Med J* 1969;i:536–40.
[3] Caranasos GJ, Stewart RB, Cluff LE. Drug-induced illness leading to hospitalisation. *JAMA* 1974:**228**;713–7.
[4] Bottiger LE, Norlander M, Strandberg I, Westerholm B. Deaths from drugs. An analysis of drug-induced deaths reported to the Swedish adverse drug reaction committee during a five-year period (1966–1970). *J Clin Pharmacol* 1974;**8–9**:401–7.
[5] Judge TG, Caird FI. *Drug treatment of the elderly patient*. London: Pitman Medical, 1978.
[6] Law R, Chalmers C. Medicines and elderly people: a general practice survey. *Br Med J* 1976;i:565–8.
[7] Christopher LJ. Patterns of prescribing in general practice. In: Woods HF, ed. *Topics in therapeutics 6*. London: Pitman Medical, 1978:1–14.
[8] Haynes RB. A critical review of the determinants of patient compliance with therapeutic regimens. In: Sackett DL, Haynes RB, eds. *Compliance with therapeutic regimens*. Baltimore: Johns Hopkins University Press, 1976: 26–39.
[9] Parkin DM, Henney CR, Quirk J, Crooks J. Deviation from prescribed drug treatment after discharge from hospital. *Br Med J* 1976;ii:686–8.
[10] Wandless I, Davie JW. Can drug compliance in the elderly be improved? *Br Med J* 1977;i:359–61.
[11] Greenblatt DJ, Allen MD. Toxicity of nitrazepam in the elderly: a report from the Boston Collaborative Drug Surveillance Program. *Br J Clin Pharmacol* 1978;**5**:407–13.
[12] Greenblatt DJ, Allen MD, Shader RI. Toxicity of high-dose flurazepam in the elderly. *Clin Pharmacol Ther* 1977;**21**:355–61.
[13] Boston Collaborative Drug Surveillance Program. Clinical depression of the central nervous system due to diazepam and chlordiazepoxide in relation to cigarette smoking and age. *N Engl J Med* 1973;**288**:277–80.
[14] Jick H, Slone D, Borda IT, Shapiro S. Efficacy and toxicity of heparin in relation to age and sex. *N Engl J Med* 1968;**279**:284–6.
[15] Lawson DH. Adverse reactions to potassium chloride. *Q J Med* 1974;**43**: 433–40.
[16] Pfeifer HF, Greenblatt DJ. Clinical toxicity of theophylline in relation to cigarette smoking. *Chest* 1978;**73**:455–9.
[17] Greenblatt DJ, Duhme DW, Allen MD, Koch-Weser J. Clinical toxicity of furosemide in hospitalised patients. A report from the Boston Collaborative Drug Surveillance Program. *Am Heart J* 1977;**94**:6–13.
[18] Lawson DH, Gloss D, Jick H. Adverse reactions to methyldopa with particular reference to hypotension. *Am Heart J* 1978;**96**:572–9.
[19] Crooks J, O'Malley K, Stevenson IH. Pharmacokinetics in the elderly. *Clin Pharmacokinet* 1976;**1**:280–96.
[20] Vestal RE. Drug use in the elderly: a review of problems and special considerations. *Drugs* 1978;**16**:358–82.
[21] Kampmann J, Siersbaek-Nielsen K, Kristensen M, Molholm Hansen J. Rapid evaluation of creatinine clearance. *Acta Med Scand* 1974;**196**:517–20.
[22] Castleden CM, George CF, Marcer D, Hallett C. Increased sensitivity to nitrazepam in old age. *Br Med J* 1977;i:10–12.
[23] Shepherd AMM, Wilson N, Stevenson IH. Warfarin sensitivity in the elderly. In: Crooks J, Stevenson IH, eds. *Drugs and the elderly*. London: Macmillan, 1979;199–209.
[24] Vestal RE, Wood AJ, Shand DG. Reduced β-adrenoceptor sensitivity in the elderly. *Clin Pharmacol Ther* 1979;**26**:181–6.
[25] Buhler FR, Burkart F, Lutold BE, Kung M, Marbet G, Pfisterer M. Antihypertensive beta blocking action as related to renin and age: a pharmacologic tool to identify pathogenetic mechanisms in essential hypertension. *Am J Cardiol* 1975;**36**:653–69.

Prescription writing

B H HARTLEY

A prescription is the prescriber's order for a particular patient or patients. This chapter, which considers only the prescription to the order of a general medical practitioner, provides general guidance, and the contents represent my views alone and in no way commit the DHSS.

Prescribers are expected to conform to an established convention when writing prescriptions, and certain legal requirements have to be observed before the pharmacist may supply the requested medicines. Supplying medicines against an incorrectly written prescription might lead to a contravention of the law by the pharmacist supplying the medicines, although it would not be a contravention by the prescriber. Therefore, it is the pharmacist's responsibility to be conversant with the law and for him to query suspected illegalities or irregularities however they arise. Legislative requirements are principally concerned to ensure authentication of the prescription and to restrict opportunities for patients to present fraudulent prescriptions for dispensing. Consequently most legislation applies to specific legal categories of medicines and requires such things as indelibility, original signature, date of prescribing, and patient's name and address. The table sets out the orders and regulations bearing on prescription writing.

TYPES OF PRESCRIPTIONS

The written prescription may be for a National Health Service or a private patient. The private patient pays for the drugs or appliances and the pharmacist's professional fee.

Writing private prescriptions

There are somewhat fewer restrictions on the prescriber in the private sector than in the NHS. To minimise the pharmacist's doubts about the authenticity of private prescriptions they should be written either on a specially printed prescription form or on the prescriber's headed notepaper. Unlike NHS prescriptions a private prescription, apart from one for Controlled Drugs, is repeatable if so marked. If marked "Repeat x times" it can be first dispensed and then repeated x times. If the prescriber writes the word "Repeat" it can be indefinitely repeated if it is not a prescription-only medicine (POM). These can be repeated only once, although even so an exception is made for oral contraceptives, which may be repeated at intervals of one month up to a maximum of six times. To avoid possible misunderstandings it is prudent to mark repeat prescriptions with the number of repeats intended.

Legal requirements bearing on prescription writing

	Regulation or order	General requirements
Nature of the prescription Doctors' terms of service	The National Health Service (General Medical and Pharmaceutical Services) Regulations 1974: SI No 160 (in Scotland 1974: SI No 506)	NHS prescriptions to be written on FP10 (GP10 in Scotland) with full signature in ink after items entered on the form. Separate form for each patient with exception in England and Wales for two or more patients in schools and institutions with over 20 residents if the doctor is responsible for 10 or more residents
Special requirements for prescription-only medicines (POM)	The Medicines (Prescription only) Order 1977: SI 2127 as amended	Prescription for POM must be indelible, have address and usual signature of practitioner, date of signature, qualifications of prescriber (that is, medical, dental, etc) Name and address of patient, age if under 12 Carbon copies with date before which prescription cannot be dispensed.
Special requirements for Controlled Drugs	The Misuse of Drugs Regulations 1973: SI 797 as amended	Prescriptions for Schedule 2 and 3 drugs must be for a single individual in ink or otherwise indelible with usual signature, no copies, name and address of patient in doctor's own handwriting, address of person issuing a private prescription Specify in doctor's own handwriting dose to be taken and in the case of preparations form and where appropriate strength of preparation, total quantity (in both words and figures) of preparation, or number in words and figures of dosage units to be supplied, or total quantity of controlled drug ordered Instalment prescriptions must have a direction specifying amount of each instalment and intervals to be observed between each dispensing. Prescriber must be in Britain, and pharmacist must be reasonably satisfied that it is the prescriber's signature Prescription cannot be dispensed before date on prescription and not later than 13 weeks afterwards
Labelling of dispensed medicines with instructions for use	The Medicines (Labelling) Regulations 1976: SI 1726	If requested by doctor on prescription form dispensed medicine shall be labelled with name of medicine, any directions for use written on prescription, and any precautions relating to use of medicine

Writing NHS prescriptions

NHS prescriptions must be written on FP10 in England and Wales and GP10 in Scotland and in accordance with the doctor's terms of service. Doctors on the Family Practitioner Committee's medical list may prescribe any drug needed for the patient's treatment as well as those appliances and chemical reagents listed in the *Drug Tariff*.

Bulk prescribing—The terms of service require that a separate FP10 or GP10 is written for each patient. In England and Wales only, however, bulk prescriptions are permissible when prescribing for two or more people in a residential school or institution in which at least 20 people reside and when the doctor is responsible for the treatment of at least 10 of the residents. Instead of the name of the patient the bulk prescription is headed with the name of the school or institution and the number of people for whom the prescriber is responsible. The range of drugs that may be prescribed in this way is limited, and the publication *Residential Homes for the Elderly*[1] provides further advice on the subject of what to prescribe.

Carbon-copies—Although repeatable prescriptions and those referring to previous ones are not permitted, up to three carbon copy FP10's are permissible for all except controlled drugs. Carbon copies should be dated with the date before which they cannot be dispensed. The doctor is required to sign the completed FP10 and each carbon copy in ink with initials or forename and surname.

ARRANGEMENT OF A PRESCRIPTION

A prescription conventionally consists of:

The patient's name and address;

The "inscription," now only occasionally preceded by the symbol Rx, which is the abbreviation for *recipe*, Latin for "take," which describes the prescribed medication;

The "subscription" preceded by *Mitte*, Latin for "send," which gives the quantity ordered or preferably the dose of the medicine and the number of doses required;

The signetur, abbreviated to *Sig*, Latin for "label," which is the prescriber's instructions to the patient including the dosage requirements which will be written on the medicine label by the pharmacist;

The prescriber's signature authenticating the prescription;

The date of prescribing;

The prescriber's name and address.

Prescription writing

Identifying the patient

The name and address of the patient should be stated, taking particular care to distinguish members of the family or common local names. The accurate address helps the pharmacist by providing a double check when issuing the dispensed items. An indication of the age of the patient guides the pharmacist when checking dilutions and dosage and in writing label instructions for use in such a way as to minimise confusion about taking or administering the medicine. NHS prescriptions for children under 12 years should state their age. Women over 60 and men over 65 will mark the back of the FP10 and so provide the pharmacist with a clue to their age.

The inscription

Drugs and appliances should always be described in English and not by Latin titles, as was formerly the case. Drugs may be described by their official (generic) name unless it is the prescriber's intention that a particular proprietary preparation should be dispensed.

A wide range of products can be prescribed, and it is imperative that the name is legible and accurately and fully describes the preparation including the required strength and dose-form where appropriate. Several preparations have similar names that can easily be confused. Lists of look-alike names are published, and a useful list was published in the *BMJ*.[2]

The subscription

Matching up of quantities—The subscription is the ordering quantity of the medicine and should be directly related to the duration of treatment. Unfortunately, most prescriptions for tablets and capsules are written in multiples of 10, whereas it could be better to prescribe a daily dose and the number of days for which treatment is required. There is a space on NHS prescription forms to facilitate ordering by days. Daily or weekly ordering is universally adopted in hospitals, and it makes particularly good sense to continue it into general practice. The advantage apart from logical prescribing of quantities is in providing the best means of balancing the patient's order when more than one item is prescribed, so giving the patient a check on whether or not they are complying with the dosage. Furthermore, as original pack dispensing becomes more common, the daily dose multiplied by the number of days treatment provides a rational basis for pack sizing. Another advantage is in overcoming wastage, particularly for patients with repeat prescriptions for more than one item where one item is consumed faster than others. Often the entirety of the order is prescribed on the repeat, although the patient needs only the replenishment of the item used most. For example, a prescription with two items both of which are often used by the patient.

Tabs "X" one twice a day send 50 tabs: this will give 25 days' supply.

Tabs "Y" one three times a day send 100: this will give 33 days' supply.

After 25 days the patient returns for a repeat prescription, although there are still eight days' treatment of Y remaining. Nevertheless, the repeat prescription is likely to reproduce the original, leading to a gradual build-up of tablets Y.

It would be much better therefore to prescribe in the following way:

Tabs X one twice a day 28 days—56 tablets will be supplied.

Tabs Y one three times a day 28 days—84 tablets will be supplied.

How to order quantities—The nature of the product needs to be taken into consideration as well as the duration of treatment. The following general advice [3] will lead to prescriptions that are both intelligible to the pharmacist and should overcome potential hazards of displaced decimal points, etc.

(1) Dose levels for solids in excess of 1 gram should be stated in multiples and fractions of 1 gram. Quantities under 1 gram should be written in milligrams—for instance, 500 mg and not 0·5 g. Similarly, quantities under 1 mg should be written in micrograms—for instance, 100 micrograms (unabbreviated) and not 0·1 mg. Where decimals are unavoidable a zero should be written in front of the decimal point, 0·5 g not ·5 g.

(2) Solid dose internal preparations, such as capsules, tablets, cachets, and suppositories, should be based on the dose and the duration of treatment. Only when it is impossible to calculate the dose, such as when a product is to be taken as the need arises, for instance, analgesics, is it necessary to state a numerical quantity to be supplied. Write the quantity in words when prescribing drugs prone to abuse; this is obligatory for Controlled Drugs.

(3) For external dose solids such as powders, dusting powders, pastes, and ointments the quantity prescribed should be selected from the range 5 g, 10 g, 15 g, 25 g, 50 g, 100 g, 200 g, 300 g, and 500 g.

(4) Liquid preparations for internal use are in doses of 5 ml for linctuses and elixirs and paediatric preparations and 10 ml for adult mixtures. A single dose of 5 ml may be better for elderly patients, who might be forgetful and unreliable about taking two spoonfuls. The pharmacist will ensure that the patient has a 5 ml teaspoon with the prescription. Drops and paediatric Digoxin elixir are an exception to the general rule, droppers or a pipette are usually associated with the preparation.

(5) The volume of oral liquid preparations should normally be sufficient to supply multiples of 10 doses—that is, 50 ml, 100 ml, 150 ml, 200 ml, 300 ml, or 500 ml.

(6) The prescribed quantity of topical preparations will depend on

the part of the body being treated, but in general large volumes, for instance, 500 ml, are suitable for treatment of the whole body, 200 ml for sizable areas such as the limbs, and 100 ml for smaller areas such as the face. Advice about topical creams and ointments is somewhat difficult because the medicine is often in an original pack that greatly determines the convenient quantity for dispensing. As a general guide small areas require quantities varying between 5 g and 15 g according to the frequency of usage, medium areas require 25–50 g, and larger areas of the body 100–200 g.

(7) Liniments are best ordered in quantities of 100 ml.

(8) Eye lotions, gargles, and mouth washes are best ordered in quantities of 200 ml.

(9) Inhalations and sprays are best ordered in quantities of 25 ml.

(10) Eye, nose, and ear drops are best ordered in quantities of 10 ml, remembering that sterile preparations should not be kept longer than one month after opening.

Signetur—the directions to be given to the patient

The directions for use are an important but often neglected component of the prescription. Properly written they could considerably aid compliance. Labelling regulations made under the Medicines Act require the pharmacist to transfer to the medicine label any instructions or directions or special notice written on the prescription itself. Unfortunately, the great majority of prescriptions are deficient in this respect, but explicit instructions would possibly lead to greater understanding by the patient as to the means of and necessity for taking the medicine. In some parts of the country prescribers have made informal arrangements with the local pharmacists so that agreed instructions appear on the labels of particular products unless the prescriber states otherwise.

The important features of instructions to be given to the patients are how and when to take the medicine and any frequently experienced side effects that may influence judgment—for instance, drowsiness, dietary restrictions, and avoidance of alcohol. Commonly used instructions need to be critically reviewed. Why write one at night if what is meant is one at bedtime; similarly one three times a day means when precisely? In the absence of clear unequivocal instructions it is not surprising that patients make up their own minds about when to take their medicine.

Some special warnings are automatically provided for specific medicaments. On a national basis warning cards are automatically given in respect of monoamine oxidase inhibitors pointing out to the patient the vital necessity of avoiding certain foods. Warning cards also exist for certain corticosteroids and anticoagulants.

The Councils of the British Medical Association and the

Pharmaceutical Society have agreed that for NHS prescriptions the name of the preparation and its strength when appropriate will appear on the medicine label unless the prescriber indicates otherwise. This arrangement does not apply when the made-up preparation has several ingredients. The name written on the label will be that used by the prescriber on the prescription. If the prescriber does not wish the name to appear on the label he need only delete the letters NP which appear on the FP10. The same applies to Controlled Drugs. Private prescriptions will not automatically be labelled NP unless the prescriber writes the letters NP alongside those items he wishes to be named on the label.

Completing and signing the prescription

Draw a diagonal line across the unused part of the form below the prescription and add initials against any altered items. The prescription is completed with the prescriber's usual signature, the date of prescribing, and the prescriber's address. (The address is preprinted on FP10 and GP10.)

PRESCRIPTION WRITING FOR CONTROLLED DRUGS

Certain safeguards have to be complied with by the prescriber to safeguard pharmacists against dispensing fraudulently written prescriptions for Controlled Drugs. The Misuse of Drugs Regulations 1973 permit only lawful dealings in Controlled Drugs, and unless the prescription conforms with the regulations the pharmacist cannot legally supply the drugs to the patient.

The prescription must:

(*a*) be in writing and signed by the person issuing it with his usual signature and dated by him;

(*b*) be indelible;

(*c*) include the address of the person issuing it;

(*d*) be complete with the patient's name and address in the doctor's own handwriting;

(*e*) give details of the dose, the dose form where appropriate, the strength and the total quantity of the preparation, and the number of dosage units to be supplied both in words as well as in figures. If for any reason these figures cannot be given the total quantity of the Controlled Drug should be stated on the prescription;

(*f*) repeatable prescriptions are not permitted for Controlled Drugs so that in the case of a prescription for a total quantity intended to be dispensed by instalments the prescription should contain a direction specifying the amount of the instalments that may be dispensed and the intervals to be observed between dispensing.

The Home Secretary has the power to waive "own handwriting"

provisions, but this is intended as a relaxation to allow the use of rubber stamps in drug treatment centres.

NHS PRESCRIPTIONS FOR APPLIANCES AND DRESSINGS

Only those appliances and dressings listed in part VI of the *Drug Tariff* are allowable on an NHS prescription. Many prescriptions for appliances incorrectly describe the article or fail to give sufficient detail; correct descriptions are given in the *Drug Tariff*.

Prescriptions for elastic hosiery should state whether a single or pair of articles is required, the name of the article—for instance anklet or thigh stockings—and the fabric—for instance one-way stretch, standard or light-weight elastic yarn or net. Comprehensive advice is given in the *Drug Tariff*.

Writing accurate prescriptions for the various stoma appliances available on the market can be difficult, and it is a help if doctors include on the prescription the reference number of the stoma appliance that the patient has had fitted.

GLOSSARY

A prescription	A written order, signed by a practitioner for a named drug.
Controlled drugs ...	Drugs listed in schedules 2 or 3 of Misuse of Drugs Regulations 1973.
Drug Tariff	Produced annually by DHSS under Reg 58 of NHS (General Medical and Pharmaceutical Services) Regulations 1974—Amended regularly as necessary throughout the year.
Listed appliances ...	Appliances including dressings listed in part VI of *Drug Tariff*. Only listed appliances may be prescribed on NHS.
Listed chemical reagents	Listed in part V of *Drug Tariff*.

REFERENCES

[1] Department of Health and Social Security. *Residential homes for the elderly*. London: HMSO, 1977.

[2] McNulty H, Spurr P. Drug names that look or sound alike. *B Med J* 1979; ii: 83

[3] *British National Formulary* London: Pharmacentical Press, 1981.

Index

Index

Index

Index

Index

Index

Index